The People's Pelvis

An All-Age, All-Gender Coloring Tour of Pelvic Health!

by Rachael Wilder

Austin, Texas 2022

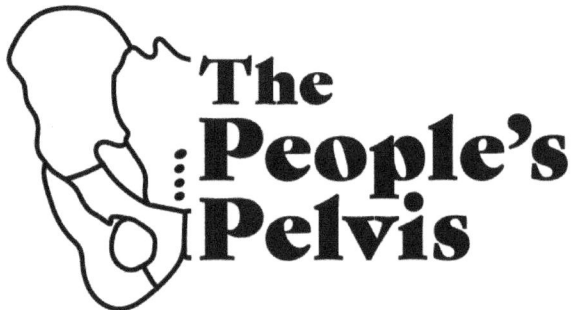

The People's Pelvis, 2nd Edition

ISBN: 978-1-7372763-0-2

www.peoplespelvis.com

On social media @ The People's Pelvis

Cover art by Noël Kalmus

Book design by Noël Kalmus and Recspec

Illustrations by Rachael Wilder and Noël Kalmus

Editing by Abe Louise Young

Table of Contents

Introducing...
Your Pelvis!

Welcome to this great and mysterious place.

The pelvis is a powerful part of you, and misunderstandings abound! Like so many others, I didn't have a great relationship with my own as a young adult. It seemed to be the source of so many discomforts, and eventually, real pathology! I believe that understanding the physiology and psychology of the workings of your pelvis can lead to lots of health and happiness... and provide an anchor if you ever need to navigate challenges therein. So, like my teachers who have come before me and those who will come after me, I am on a mission to help people learn and understand how their bodies work before issues arise, and to give you encouragement when they do!

In the whole wide world, this information is very spread out either in sound-bites, or not generally geared towards regular folk, and can be rather boring to read cover-to-cover. I mean, piles of books and articles are great when you want to dive deep, but you are busy people, right?! I wanted to create a fun way to learn the basics. Hence, an educational coloring book was born! Let it serve as a primer to pelvic health, so that if and when anything arises that you need to address, you have a base to work from as you research and learn more.

Another goal is to foster respect for our amazing bodies and the amazing bodies of everyone around us. Some of this information will be specific to your body, and some not, but I believe that learning about all of our bodies could change the way we see ourselves and each other for the better! So, take a seat, break out the coloring supplies, ask questions, talk with friends and trusted allies, and enjoy this coloring tour of the pelvis!

*__Bolded and italicized__ words are defined in the glossary of terms in the back of the book.

The People's Pelvis

The human pelvis is made up of 3 bones and 3 joints.

The two biggest bones, one on each side, are divided up into three sections: The **ilium** is the largest part, and the one we commonly think of as our hips. The **ischium** is at the bottom and is the attachment site for many of our leg muscles. The **pubic bone** is in the front. The two sides of the pubic bone come together in the center at a joint called the **pubic symphysis**.

In the back of your pelvis, the two ilium bones join the third bone of the pelvis, the sacrum. These three bones join together at the two sacroiliac joints (aka 'SI joints'), one on each side.

The ischium (the ones at the very bottom of your bottom) are your '**sitz bones**', or **ischial tuberosities**. As the nickname implies, these are the bones you feel under you while you sit! At least you should...frequent rolling of the pelvis so that you are sitting back on your sacrum is no good! I know, you feel so chill with your feet up on that table, but we will get into what happens with these misalignments in a bit.

The pelvis is structured to house and protect your pelvic organs, muscles, nerves, and blood vessels. It also provides attachment sites for the muscles that move you and groove you! If we didn't have a skeleton, we would just be a big pile of pulsating mush going nowhere slowly! Of course, there are many variations on how people are born or end up in life, and the skeleton is no stranger to this. We can adapt to less limbs, more or less vertebrae, diverse bone structure, and many variations of body structure and function pretty darn well! The disability rights community teaches us that what might look like a dysfunction to one person is actually another person's superpower![1]

Now let's talk about bones. Our bones serve multiple functions:

They protect our organs from trauma. This is really a balancing act between protection and the freedom to move. If we were completely covered in a layer of bone, we would be safe in some ways, but unable to move. We also need to adapt to changes in body structure, such as growth and pregnancy.

They anchor our muscles. Individual muscles need a place to attach, so they can function. The part of a muscle that attaches to a bone is called a **tendon**. Both ends of each muscle thicken, forming a strong tendon to affix to the bone.

They stabilize and move us. Bones are like the 'tent poles' that give us form and the levers that allow us to move. Along with muscles, ligaments and cartilage, they form different kinds of joints to allow even more complex movement! They are pretty darn rad.

But bones are also actually somewhat like organs too! There are vital things happening inside them that keep us alive! We produce blood cells in the marrow of our bones, plus they store minerals and energy. They're more than they're cracked up to be...HA!!

Who'da thunk?

Bones have their own circulatory system, and it's important to keep them healthy, even though it seems like they are just sitting there being bones! Bone density decreases with age, especially after menopause or age seventy.[2] The reduction in the hormone estrogen after menopause is directly linked to a decrease in bone density, which is why osteoporosis is more common in our elder family. With age, the body uses the minerals stored in the bones, which changes their strength and resilience. Calcium and vitamin D are important allies in keeping your bones healthy, so eat those greens and get a little sunshine every day, and use supplements if your levels are off. Regular, gentle exercise and hydration are also imperative ways to keep those bones from breakin'! Walking and light weight-bearing exercises are the best for bones and joints!

The shape of the bony pelvis is perfectly designed to allow the passage of nerves, arteries and veins so they get where they need to go safely. It also protects the very important functions happening within. We are going to explore all of the amazing functions happening inside and around the pelvis, but for now...

ALL HAIL THE BONY PELVIS!

THE PELVIS!

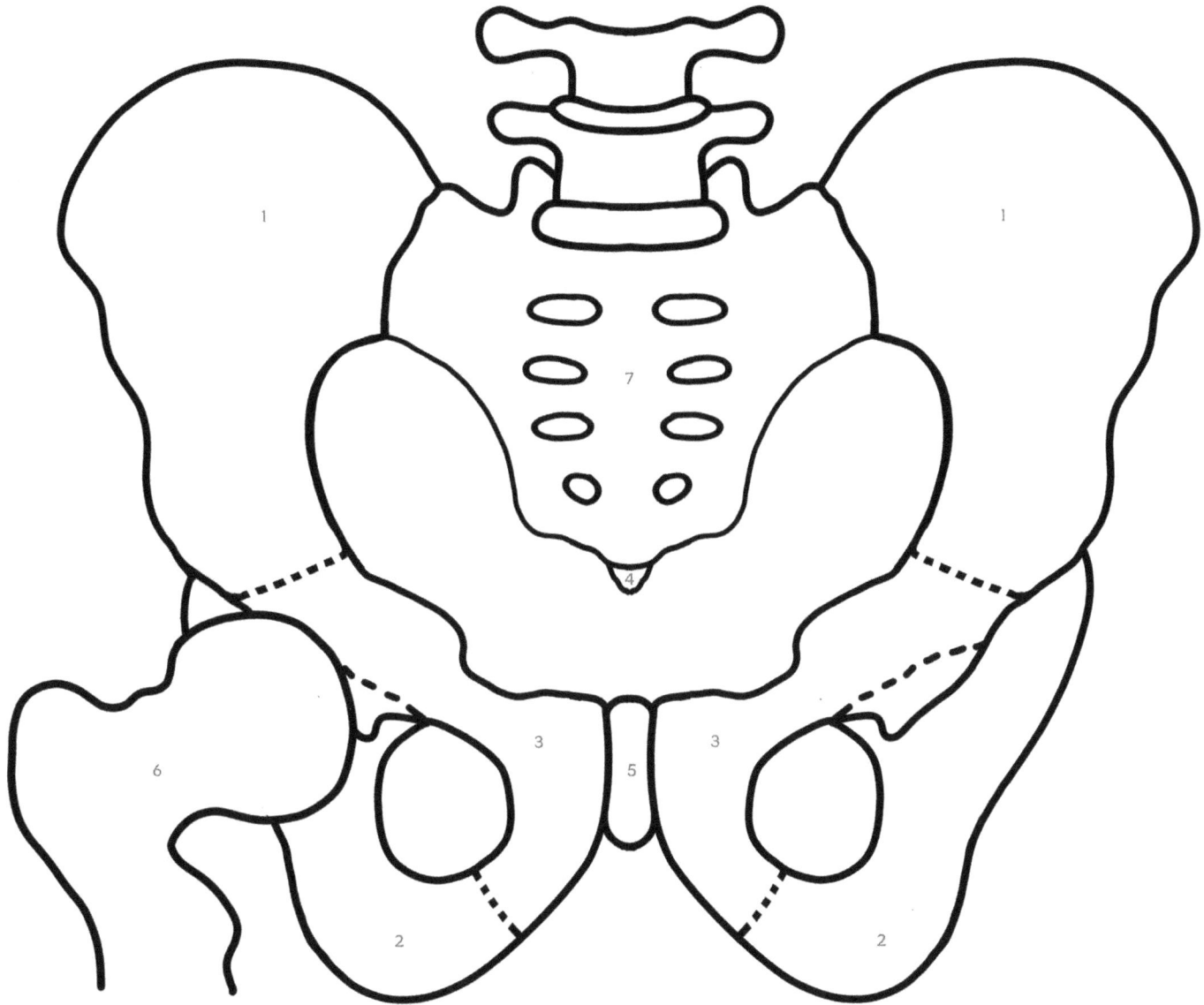

1. ILIUM
2. ISCHIUM
3. PUBIC BONE
4. TAILBONE/COCCYX
5. PUBIC SYMPHYSIS
6. FEMUR
7. SACRUM

The Bony Pelvis . . . from Behind!

The flipside of your pelvis. Also known as *'your behind.'*

At the center is your **sacrum** (aka the 'sacred' or 'holy' bone). Long thought to be the center, hub or anchor of all movement, it has been a very revered bone over the ages and deserves the props! Cultures and religions around the world have held this bone in high esteem.[3]

When you were born, your sacrum was actually 5 **spinal vertebrae**, but during childhood and young adulthood, they fuse into one bone—a process which is completed by age 26![4] A line of holes (called 'foramen') run down each side of this bone, allowing nerves and blood vessels to pass through that help run your pelvic organs and muscles. Isn't it interesting that this bone not only fuses, but leaves perfectly symmetrical openings for the passage of nerves and blood! Evolution is so smart!

Did I mention that your body is AMAZING?

The sacrum is at the very bottom of your spinal column, with your lumbar, thoracic and cervical vertebrae above it. The joint between the lowest lumbar (low back) vertebrae (L5) and the top of the sacrum (S1) is referred to as L5/S1 (*obvs*). This can be a common place for pain or injury. Remember when we talked about sitting on your sitz bones? This is that. The weird positions we get into when what we really need is a break...can break us!

The base of the sacrum is punctuated by your tailbone, or **coccyx**. Hard falls on the tailbone or sacrum hurt! If you've ever had to sit on a donut pillow, *you know*. Make sure to address any injury here with a physical therapist, professional massage therapist, chiropractor, or see a doctor if you are having ongoing pain.

Here we also see the **ligaments** that hold the bones together. Ligaments go from bone-to-bone (whereas tendons go from muscle-to-bone). They provide a great deal of stability to all of the joints of your body. These layers of ligaments cover all sides of your SI joints (right to left, inside and outside), as well as all of the joints of the body (in different configurations and amounts). If it weren't for ligaments, we would be a mess! They help keep joints going in the right direction...because the wrong direction hurts. By nature, they have less blood supply than muscles, which means they take longer to heal and require special treatment during the healing process. What works to heal a muscle could actually be bad for an injured ligament, so getting an accurate diagnosis is key! Injured ligaments don't like to be stretched during a good portion of their healing. Rest-is-best during the process, which can be very difficult if it is a high-demand joint, like a shoulder or a knee. We do the best we can, but it can be a long haul, so get yourself some good advice!

The sacroiliac joints can also be common places of pain due to poor posture, injury or repetitive stress. While we may not feel the pain for many years, it is important to keep our joints mobile and healthy to avoid difficult-to-fix issues with age. Too much of *anything* (sitting, jumping, lifting, standing, running, et al.) is not healthy for your bones, joints, muscles...or the rest of your body! Mix it up! *Move it, people!*

All of these structures are serving and supporting multiple functions of your body, so keeping them healthy and addressing injury and dysfunction has many benefits. Seek quality advice and qualified assistance. Advocating for yourself is a skill you will use forever, and sometimes it takes a few tries. Don't let anyone talk over you or disregard your questions or concerns. Find professionals who will actually listen...they *do* exist!

I also recommend making a plan before you go to *any* type of doctor or practitioner:

- Document all of the symptoms as best as you can.

- If possible, ask your family for a full history. This one is so important! Our families often don't think to mention lots of things! And if the form doesn't cover what you are experiencing, write it in!

- Research your issue so you know what questions to ask.

- Make a list of questions and expect them to be answered.

- Decide what you want the outcome to be and discuss how to get there.

It is very common for a strange, mysterious fog to descend over our heads at these appointments and make us forget everything we meant to say or ask, and also what we hear, so bring it all with you and write down what they say...or bring a friend to join you. Support can be priceless in these moments!*

*I have no evidence-based research to back this up, but *it's a thing!*

You are the one you've been waiting for!

THE PELVIS!

...FROM BEHIND

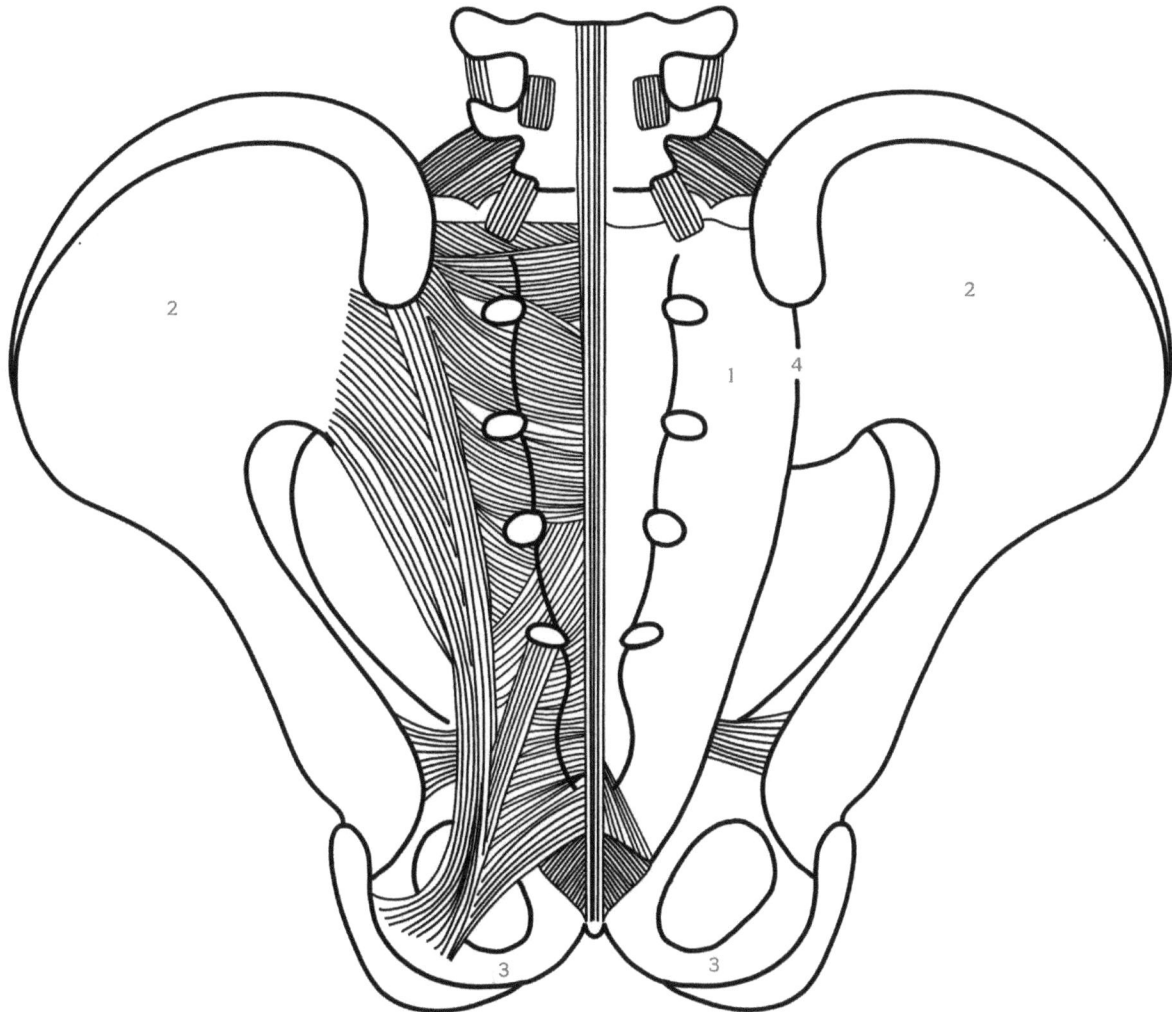

LAYERS OF LIGAMENTS

1. SACRUM   3. ISCHIUM
2. ILIUM   4. SI JOINT

Made of Muscle

Here is your bony pelvis with *some* of the muscle attachment sites marked on it. There are a *ton* of muscles attached to your pelvis! Anchoring movement above, movement below, movement within...this is one of the power centers of your strategically designed body!

While you might want to sit down and memorize each and every one of these muscles and bony landmarks (ok, you probably don't), there *is* one thing I'd like you to take away:

Muscles pull on bones!

Ideally, you have perfectly balanced muscle contractions and releases, keeping you moving throughout your days with grace and ease. Each movement you make is a full orchestra of choreographed action! But chronically tight muscles or groups of muscles pull on bones, which changes the shape of your skeleton. This has an effect on *other* muscles, nerve and organ function, and ultimately *everything*!

SO DRAMATIC.

Imagine for a moment: one tight right hamstring (the muscles in the back of the thigh). Pulling down on that right hip bone, it changes the orientation of the bone, as well as the tension on the SI joint, the spine and their ligaments. Your body is super smart and will try to stabilize you by tightening other muscles, creating a *tension pattern*. This is no biggie if it's short lived. But uncorrected for months, years, or even decades, it can create layers of problems as you try to live your best life—and who has time for that? Pain and discomfort are messages from your body.

Modern life is killing us, people! Our pelvises don't want any part of it!

I'm just sayin'. Sitting at school, sitting at home, sitting with friends, sitting alone...this is not an ode to sitting, but a rally against it! I protest, and so do our bodies!

I'm not going to lie...I speak from the experience of doing it wrong! And I sometimes still do. But once the body starts talking, it can be like the chattiest chatterbox around, for better *and* worse. I try to listen, and rue the days I don't!

Too much drama?

Regular *gentle* cardio, walking, *gentle* yoga/stretching, ergonomics, bodywork, stress reduction efforts of all types... MOVEMENT! If you consider all of the things you do repetitively (sitting at school, standing at work, guitar playing, sports, couch potatoing, drawing, video games, texting, computer work, carrying children, cooking up a storm), those tension patterns need to be undone so they don't turn into stone.

Don't be a stone.

A common mental trap people fall into is 'all or nothing' thinking when it comes to exercise (and everything else). Somehow, if we aren't training for a marathon, we're failing at health. Walking for 20 minutes/day-ish can have a profound impact on both physical and emotional health. Alternate with some yoga, light weight training, frisbee, bicycling, or whatever inspires you will be setting yourself up for long-term success.

Of course, as with anything else, you *can* overdo it with exercise, too. It's no better than *under* doing it! I have seen countless clients whose over-exercising is keeping them stuck in pain, tension and anxiety. Your body needs recovery time, and generally to not take things quite so seriously. Find something that makes your *soul* slow *down*!

A 2018 study published by the National Center for Biotechnology Information (NCBI) states, "The prevalence rate of exercise addiction was 4.0% in school athletes, 8.7% in fitness attendees, and 21% in patients with eating disorders. Exercise addiction was associated with feelings of guilt when not exercising, ignoring pain and injury, and higher levels of body dissatisfaction."[5]

Are you pickin' up what I'm puttin' down? Be balanced like the Buddha.

Your body is a temple...worship!

MUSCLE ATTACHMENTS

FRONT

BACK

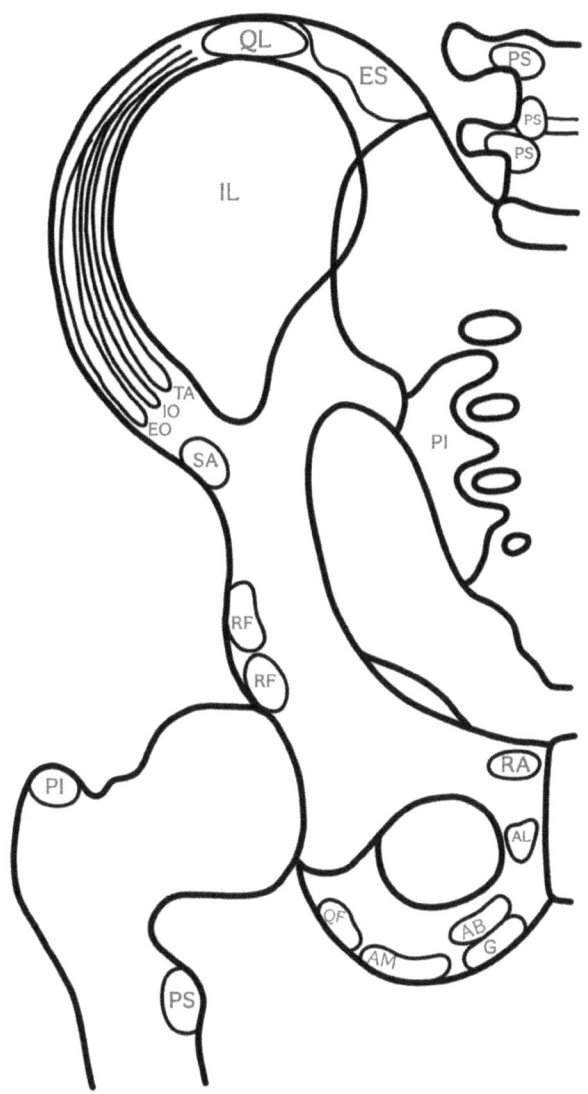

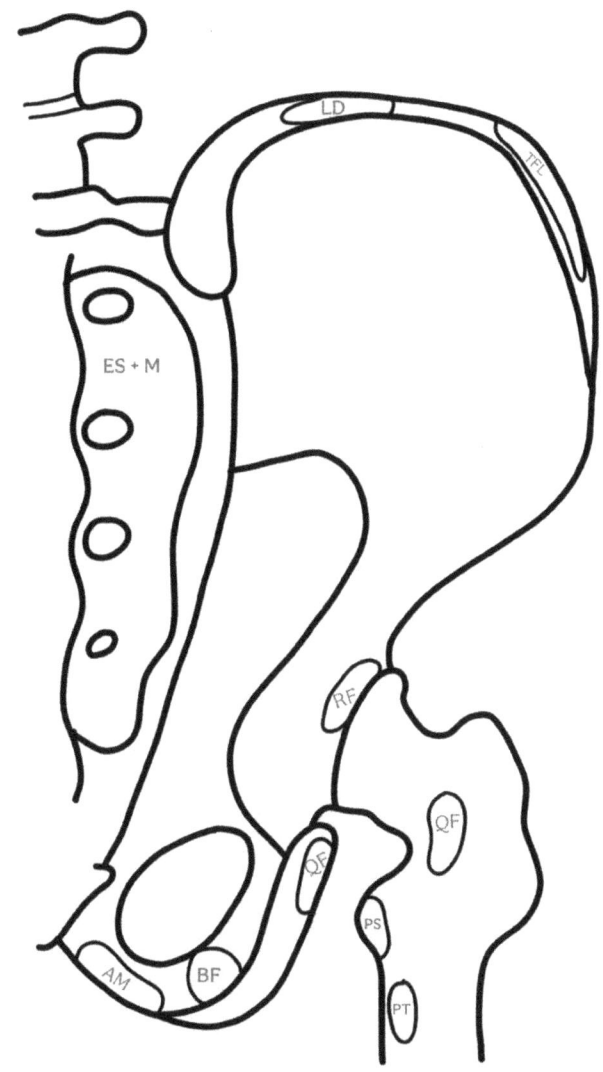

BACK MUSCLES:

Latissimus dorsi **(LD)**
Erector spinae **(ES)** + Multifidi **(M)**
Quadratus lumborum **(QL)**

ABDOMINAL MUSCLES:

External obliques **(EO)** + Internal obliques **(IO)**
Rectus abdominis **(RA)** + Transverse abdominis **(TA)**

LEG MUSCLES:

Rectus femoris **(RF)** + Biceps femoris **(BF)**
Adductor magnus **(AM)** brevis **(AB)** + longus **(AL)**
Quadratus femoris **(QF)**
Gracilis **(G)** + Tensor fasciae latae **(TFL)**
Sartorius **(SA)**

CORE MUSCLES:

Iliopsoas **(PS)** + Iliacus **(IL)**
Piriformis **(PI)** + Pectineus **(PT)**

Whoa. My Pelvis Has a Floor?

Yes, it does! It also has walls, which together form the pelvic bowl! *What the what?!*

Now that you've seen the bones that form the outside of your pelvis, and you understand how muscles relate to bones, we're ready to get down to the nitty-gritty. The pelvic floor muscles are performing very important and delicate tasks!

Your pelvic floor has different layers, and each layer is focused on different functions. There is some overlap, but let's break it down like this:[6]

The 1st layer (or the outermost) is referred to as the sexual layer. These muscles (and the nerves that control them) allow your sexual self to *express itself*...if you know what I mean. Both physical function and emotions play a role in how well these muscles and nerves do or do not work.[7] They don't just take orders down there! And sometimes they 'work' at surprising and unexpected times! Addressing your stress level is as important as learning what is happening on a physical level. We will learn about the hormones of stress and the psychology of sexuality later, but they are powerful!

The 2nd layer is called the sphincter layer (or urogenital diaphragm). These muscles control the release (or withholding) of bodily waste, commonly referred to as #1 and #2. Pretty important, right?! Lots of life events can affect these sphincters or the stuff that run them, such as childbirth, chronic constipation, scar tissue from injury or surgery, or chronic tension and stress.

The 3rd layer (or the innermost) is the supportive layer, or pelvic diaphragm. This is what is generally meant by the term 'pelvic floor'. These muscles give a supportive base to your pelvis and its contents, preventing organ prolapse (descent) and resisting intra-abdominal pressure. They also support the function of the other layers of the pelvis and act as a web of musculature connecting the bones of the pelvis. In true muscle group fashion, they allow movement, but resist hyperextension, or too much movement (which can cause injury).

Pretty radical, huh?

When the choreography of all of these muscles is on-point, which it mostly is, the pelvis is *fabulous*! Injury or dysfunction in this area can result in kidney, urinary, digestive, reproductive, sexual and other pain or function related issues...and nobody wants that!! On the flipside, when all of these muscles work together well, life is good!

Luckily, there are experts for *everything*, including physical therapists who specialize in pelvic floor health, doctors who specialize in **urogenital** health, yoga and exercises for the pelvic floor, breathing for the pelvic floor, psychotherapists who help you understand your mind/heart/body connection and how to communicate about it with your partners...it's a thing! Since many physical issues involve a combination of muscles that are too tight and also too weak or not firing well, make sure your solution is helping. There is an exercise called a kegel, which has been popularized to strengthen the pelvic floor...but what happens to the muscles that are too tight? They get tighter. Kegels are easy to do wrong and are often not the first place to get relief.[8]

You will definitely receive advice that is not actually what you need in your lifetime, so give it a go, and if it doesn't work, move along! A good health practitioner won't take it personally. They will be dynamic enough to come up with a different approach or refer you to another person.

Also, suffering through it is so yesterday.

Let's try an exercise. Yes, I want you to slow down and do a thing!

Find a chair, ideally a relatively firm one. Sit with your feet flat on the floor and your spine upright but relaxed. No slumping into the back of the chair.

Take three deep breaths. As you exhale, relax any tension you might be holding.

Feel the sensation of your 'sitz bones' on the chair's surface. Adjust your pelvis if you can't.

Feel your breath expanding downwards into the chair, the floor, and the earth as you inhale and let everything relax as you exhale. Take three deep breaths.

Now imagine a ribbon going from the tip of your tailbone, up through your spine, your skull, and up into the sky. Take three deep breaths.

Imagine yourself breathing in and out of your pelvic floor and up away into the sky, alternately, letting all tensions dissolve as you maintain an easy, aligned posture.

Relax. Breathe.

This is a great way to relax, check your posture, and help release any conscious or unconscious tension. Try it periodically throughout the day. Let it be sweet relief!

PELVIC FLOOR!

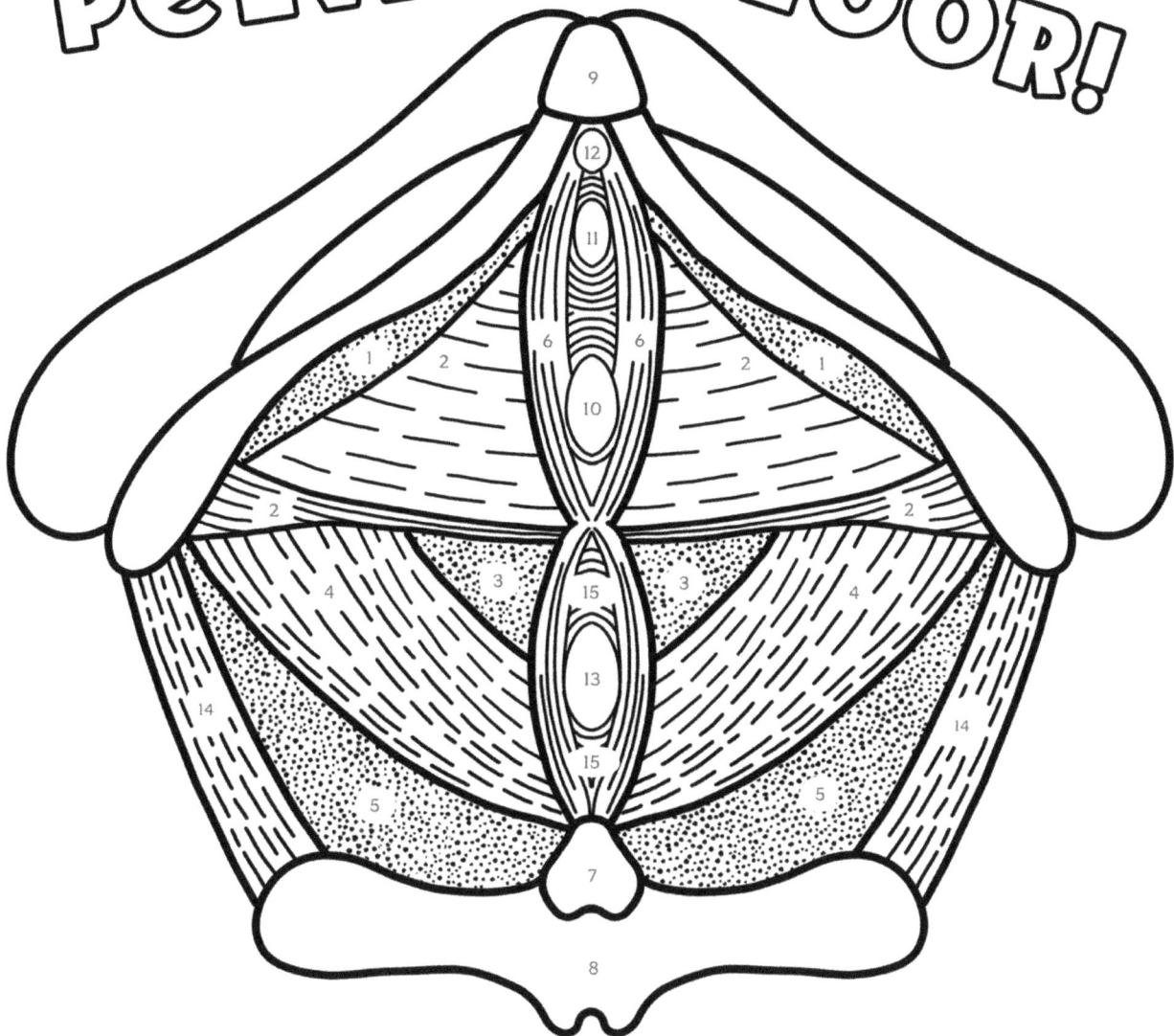

1. ISCHIOCAVERNOSUS
2. TRANSVERSE PERINEALS
3. PUBOCOCCYGEUS
4. ILIOCOCCYGEUS
5. COCCYGEUS
6. BULBOSPONGIOSUS
7. COCCYX   14. SACROTUBEROUS LIGAMENT
8. SACRUM

9. PUBIC BONE
10. VAGINA
11. URETHRA
12. CLITORIS
13. ANUS
15. ANAL SPHINCTERS

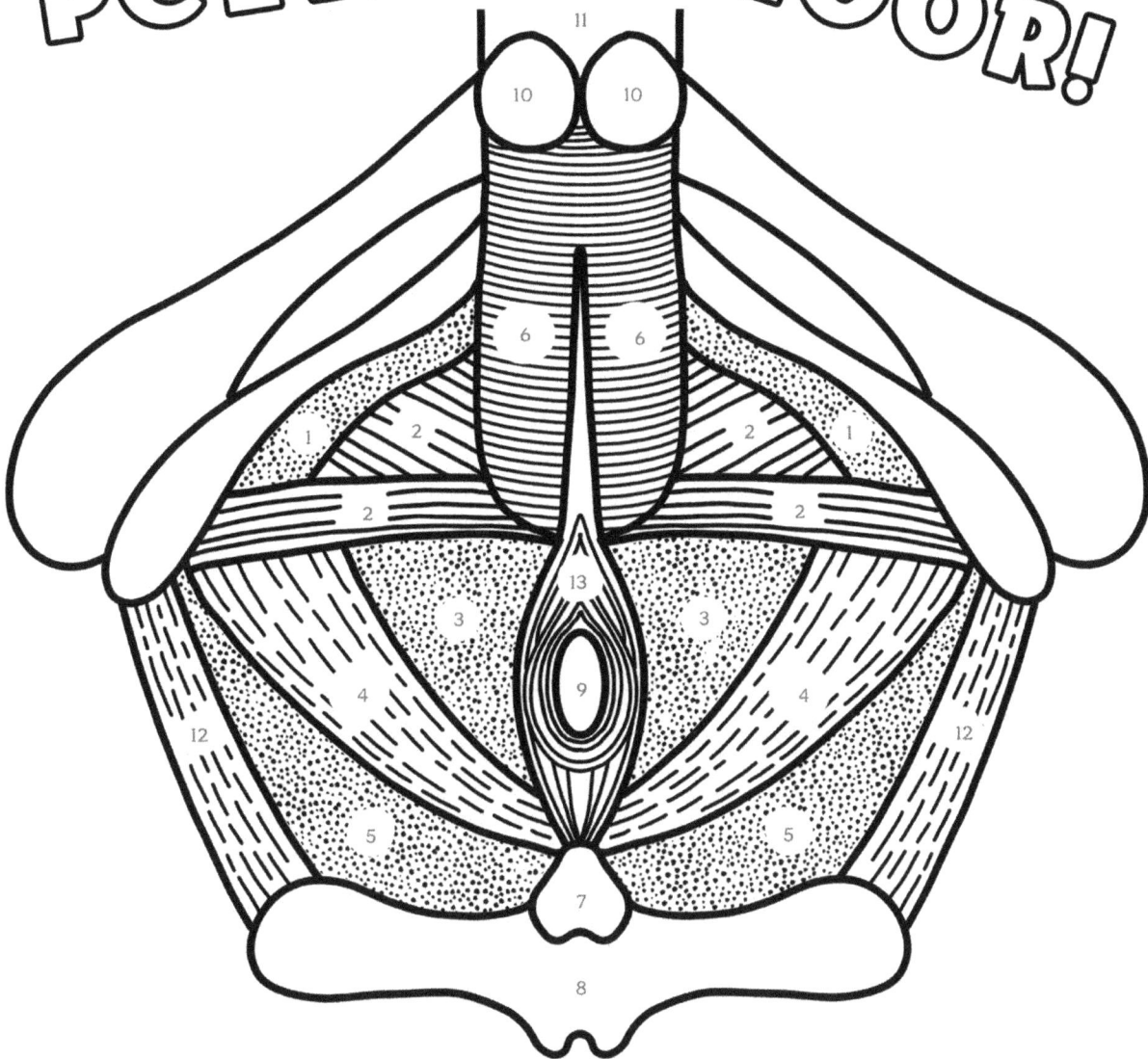

PELVIC FLOOR!

1. ISCHIOCAVERNOSUS
2. TRANSVERSE PERINEALS
3. PUBOCOCCYGEUS
4. ILIOCOCCYGEUS
5. COCCYGEUS
6. BULBOSPONGIOSUS
7. COCCYX
8. SACRUM
9. ANUS
10. TESTES
11. PENIS
12. SACROTUBEROUS LIGAMENT
13. ANAL SPHINCTERS

So ... What?!

The psoas muscle.

Pronounced *so-azz*. You've got two. Together, the psoas major and minor form the 'Iliopsoas.' The Greek translation is 'muscle of the loins.' Make all the jokes you want, but this muscle is powerful and sensitive...and could definitely take you in a fight! Mostly because it's attached to the *inside* of your lumbar spine, so when it's unhappy, it's got a direct line to pain.

There is a whole book written about the psoas. More than one, in fact. An important aspect of the structure of this muscle is that it is *jam* packed with nerves. Liz Koch (who wrote the aforementioned *Psoas Book*[9]) likens it to an organ because of its neurological sensitivity and function. She has a lot to say about the emotional and energetic intelligence of this important muscle.

I like to think of it as a sort of *emotional sonar*. It's deep within the core of your body, full of nerves, and connects your core to your legs. Emotional stress often causes a **primal** tension in this area, and the psoas leads the way. It seems to know when we're holding on to our emotions, and sense when we don't feel right. It has been said that our oldest trauma resides in the pelvis. Learning stretches and stress-relief techniques can have a profound effect on this muscle, especially if you have low back, hip or pelvic pain, or just a whole lotta stress.

Your psoas (one on each side) starts at the inside of your **lumbar spine** and descends into your hip where it runs alongside another major hip muscle, the **iliacus**. From there, it heads down through your pelvis and attaches to a spot on the inside of your femur (thigh) bone. Given the shape of it, the posture that keeps it in a shortened position is sitting. Muscles that spend their days being short start to resist being long!

When you have been sitting for a couple of hours and your psoas muscles are all comfy being short, and you stand up and say, 'Hey psoas, be long!', sometimes they protest! They can pull inward on your low back and rotate your femur into a funny (not-so-funny) position, causing tension and pain. Five, ten, twenty-plus years of that and they could get very angry (wouldn't you?!). Modern life has even very small children in crunched up, contorted positions using devices of some form or another, so those years add up quickly!

Yoga* and stretching can go a long way in helping these muscles release, so find a good source of instruction, ideally in person or one-on-one with someone who has a lot of experience and can guide you without pushing you into more pain. Your body knows!

You've only got two psoas...don't cross 'em, or they'll cross you!

I have included two other muscles, the *piriformis* and the *coccygeus*, both of which get cranky with inactivity or too much of anything.

The piriformis is the largest of a set of hip rotators, and it does a lot of bracing during movement or stress. If you've ever had a massage, it is one of those deeply relaxing muscles to have released, and you can emulate that experience at home with a tennis ball sunk into just the right spot. One of the most dramatic roles the piriformis performs takes place during pregnancy...whoa, they get tight just trying to keep it all together down there!

The coccygeus, while not technically one of the pelvic floor muscles, is closely related and bridges the larger pelvic muscles with the smaller, more intricate functions of the pelvic floor muscles. As the name implies, it's attached to the coccyx, or tailbone, so if you have an injury to your tailbone, releasing it can provide relief and allow the bone to heal and hopefully shift back to its ideal position.

*Yoga, along with many cultural practices, has been popularized in the west as a workout routine, but a true yoga practice involves not only the asanas (physical yoga poses), but also meditation and chanting, breathing practices, spiritual study and engaging with the community in service.

It's good to notice how pop culture takes and grossly oversimplifies things, leaving out aspects that create true health in ourselves, our families and our communities. Sometimes this 'taking' crosses over into cultural appropriation in its level of disrespect by profiting from an edited version and not paying homage to its roots, supporting its original practitioners or ignoring the plight of the people from whence it came. There is a *lot* to learn in this realm, so let's just commit to being aware, evolving as we go, and taking action in all the ways we can.

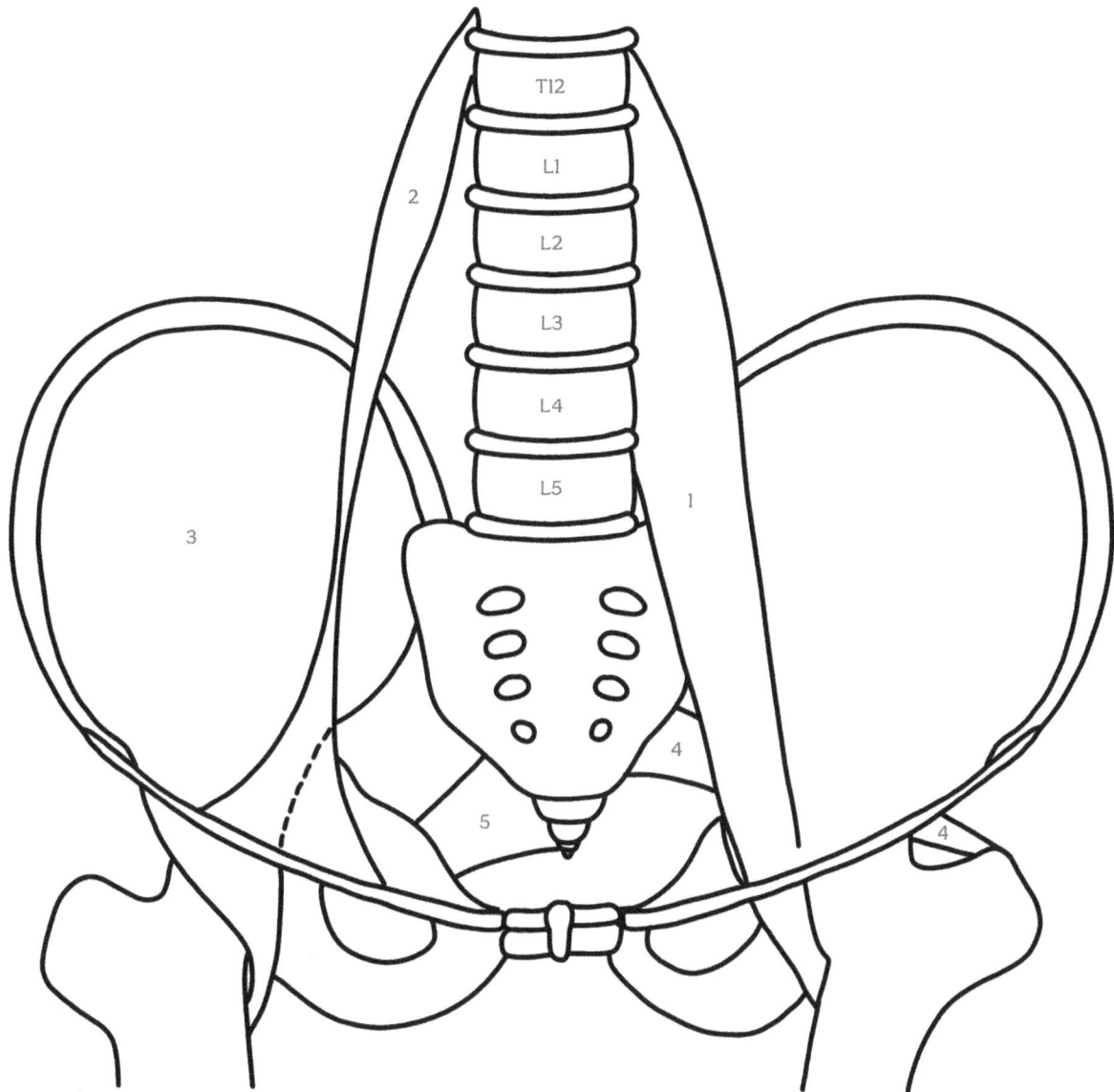

SO... WHAT?!

ILIOPSOAS: 3. ILIACUS
1. MAJOR 4. PIRIFORMIS
2. MINOR 5. COCCYGEUS

On Breathing

This jellyfish-shaped muscle is your diaphragm! I know we've used that word before to describe muscles of your pelvis, but this one most commonly bears the name. Technically it's your 'respiratory diaphragm.'

When you inhale, filling your lungs with air, the diaphragm flattens out toward your pelvis, and then rises back up into its umbrella shape when you exhale.

A healthy diaphragm not only allows you to take full breaths, but keeps the innermost parts of you moving, acting as a massage to the gut, and helping to move *lymphatic fluid* throughout your body.

The *lymphatic system* is part of your circulatory system and works to remove *cellular waste* and *pathogens* and take them to the *lymph nodes* to *destroy them*! It does other things, but is a main component of your immune system, and it's awesome.

The back of the diaphragm attaches all the way down at your lumbar spine, so we can actually relax our backs by taking some deep breaths! Chronic tension in the diaphragm can contribute to overall muscular tension in the shoulders, rib cage, neck and spine. You also want to think about the structures that pass *through* it (**the esophagus, the vena cava and the aorta**).

Tension around these structures can affect their function, which can even result in acid reflux (indigestion), or **GERD**.[10]

Breathing is something we *have* to do, but we sure are good at doing it as little as possible! Computer work is a very common situation where people barely breathe. Our upper abdomen is already somewhat tight from supporting our position, so the diaphragm is set up to fly under the radar, so to speak. Try setting an alarm on your computer or phone to remind you to take some full breaths, and you will feel the level of tension followed by relief, for real!

I'm not calling your diaphragm a slacker, but it sure does need reminding!

Remember when I said the psoas is kind of like an emotional sonar taking readings of the safety of your surroundings? I like to think of the diaphragm as an *emotional radar*...same concept with similar effects. Your breathing definitely changes when there is danger. You are actually designed that way. If you are being chased by a predator, you need extra oxygen to your brain and muscles to get you to safety, so you breathe more shallowly and quickly. The energy that usually goes to non-essential (for escape) functions like digestion and elimination get diverted to the ones that get you going fast! But you are *not* designed to keep this fight/flight/freeze mode on all of the time.[11] If modern life is restricting your diaphragms function on the daily, what impact is it having on your emotions and stress level, and vice-versa? How much of our emotional tension is reinforced by a tight diaphragm?

"Shallow breathing doesn't just make stress a response, it makes stress a habit our bodies, and therefore, our minds, are locked into," says John Luckovich, an Integrative Breathwork facilitator in Brooklyn, New York.

Long-term shallow breathing can seriously affect our health. According to Luckovich, the chronic stress that is associated with shallow breathing results in lower amounts of lymphocyte, a type of white blood cell that helps to defend the body from invading organisms, and lowers the amounts of proteins that signal other immune cells.

The body is then susceptible to contracting acute illnesses, aggravating pre-existing medical conditions, and prolonging healing times. Shallow breathing can turn into panic attacks, cause dry mouth and fatigue, aggravate respiratory problems, and is a precursor for cardiovascular issues.

This breathing pattern also creates tension in other parts of the body and can lead to a lot of everyday problems. When we breathe with our chests, we use the muscles in our shoulders, necks, and chests to expand our lungs, which can result in neck pain, headaches, and an increased risk of injury. Our shoulders slump forward and our posture changes as well."

~ Rachael Rifkin for Headspace.com

When in doubt, take three deep breaths.

Breath is life...and it's free!

BREATHE

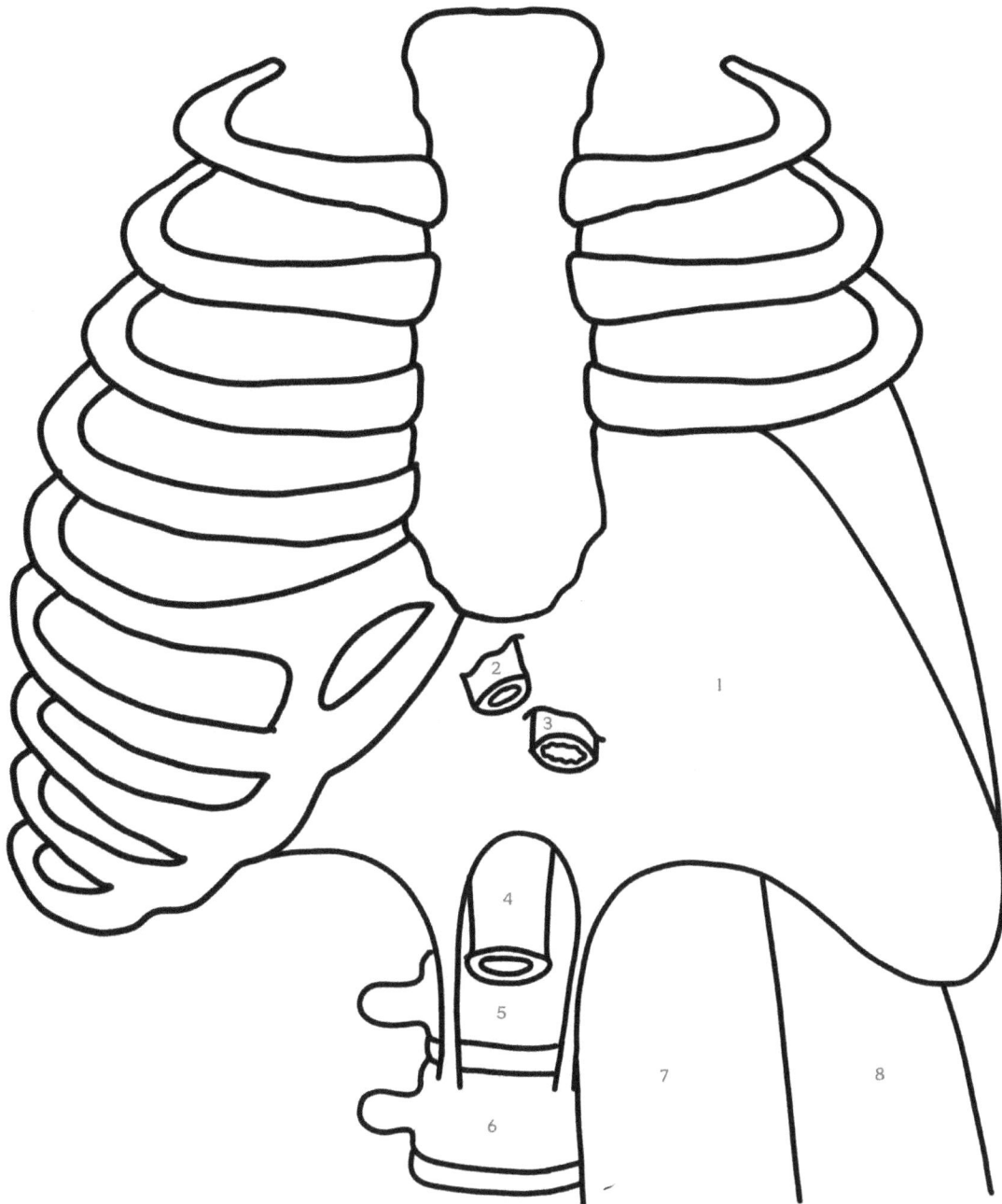

1. DIAPHRAGM
2. VENA CAVA
3. ESOPHAGUS
4. AORTA

5. LUMBAR L2
6. LUMBAR L3
7. PSOAS MAJOR
8. QUADRATUS LUMB.

You've Got Nerve!

The human nervous system is complex! But we're going to break it down into bite-sized morsels of scientific goodness. Here are the main parts:

- **The Central Nervous System (CNS):** The brain and spinal cord.

- **The Peripheral Nervous System (PNS):** A network of nerves that connect your organs, muscles and senses back to the CNS.

  ◎ **The Somatic Nervous System (SNS):** A subdivision of the PNS *generally* responsible for voluntary actions, such as whistling, winking, or reaching for a glass of water.

  ◎ **The Autonomic Nervous System (ANS):** A subdivision of the PNS *generally* responsible for the involuntary, or automatic actions, such as heart rate, metabolism, and blinking.

    • **The Sympathetic Nervous System:** A subdivision of the ANS responsible for those 'fight, flight or freeze' moments; increased heart rate, breathing and brain activity...all designed for those high-intensity times!

    • **The Parasympathetic Nervous System:** A subdivision of the ANS responsible for maintaining (or returning us to) a state of 'rest and digest', or chill time. Our bodies' energy can focus on those functions that keep us running long-term, now that we've escaped the predator or caught the prey!

    • **The Enteric Nervous System:** The nervous system of the gut. Influenced by the sympathetic and parasympathetic systems, but working independently via neurotransmitters to regulate the function of the gastrointestinal system. Also called the 'second brain' because it works independently and functions similarly to the central nervous system.

Put those definitions of the sympathetic and parasympathetic systems in your back pocket. They have grand implications for your health as it relates to stress.

Now let's get into what and why all of this matters. It's good to remember that if you are experiencing pain or sensation, it might actually be coming from somewhere else. Let's look at a short list of which nerves control what (heads up: there is overlap!):

A. Cranial nerves have a role in the function of the scalp, brain, eyes, ears, nose, mouth, vocal cords, neck muscles, shoulders, heart, lungs, diaphragm, colon and more.

B. Cervical nerves help run the scalp, neck, shoulders, arms, hands, esophagus, heart, lungs, diaphragm and more.

C. Thoracic nerves help control blood supply to the head; help run the brain, eyes, heart, lungs, gallbladder, liver, diaphragm, stomach, spleen, kidneys, small intestine, appendix and more.

D. Lumbar nerves help innervate the uterus, large intestine, buttocks, groin, other reproductive structures, colon, thighs, knees, sciatic nerve, and more.

E. Sacral nerves are connected to the buttocks, reproductive structures, bladder, prostate, sciatic nerve, lower legs, feet, rectum and more.

While it would take an injury to the spinal cord to affect organ function in a major way, even compression and chronic inflammation can create pain and dysfunction far from the source.[12] An example is sciatic nerve pain. The sciatic nerve originates in the sacral plexus (or bundle of nerves). One on each side, it runs down into the buttocks, under (and sometimes through!) the piriformis muscle, and down the back of the leg. People commonly feel the pain either at the piriformis, or in the thigh or calf. If you focus treatment on those areas only, you might get some relief, but the compression around the nerve root (via the spine) needs to be addressed.

Because we are focusing mostly on pelvic health, I want to highlight a very special nerve...the pudendal nerve. Originating from the sacral plexus, this nerve is in charge of sensation to the sexual organs, as well as function of the anus and urethra, which we want functioning well! Even long-term straining due to chronic constipation and muscle tension from emotional stress can affect this nerve![13]

Damage to the pudendal nerve can sometimes happen during childbirth, but keep in mind that deep injuries to the pelvis from events such as being kicked in the groin, breaking a bone of the pelvis, especially the sacrum, falling hard on the crossbar of a bicycle and other common injuries can cause nerve injury or damage, so be careful with yourselves and each other! I'm not trying to cry wolf here; every time you injure yourself, it's not a big emergency. You are strong, resilient, self-healing magicians so just breathe and pay attention to your body—it speaks the truth!

NERVES ARE EVERYWHERE!

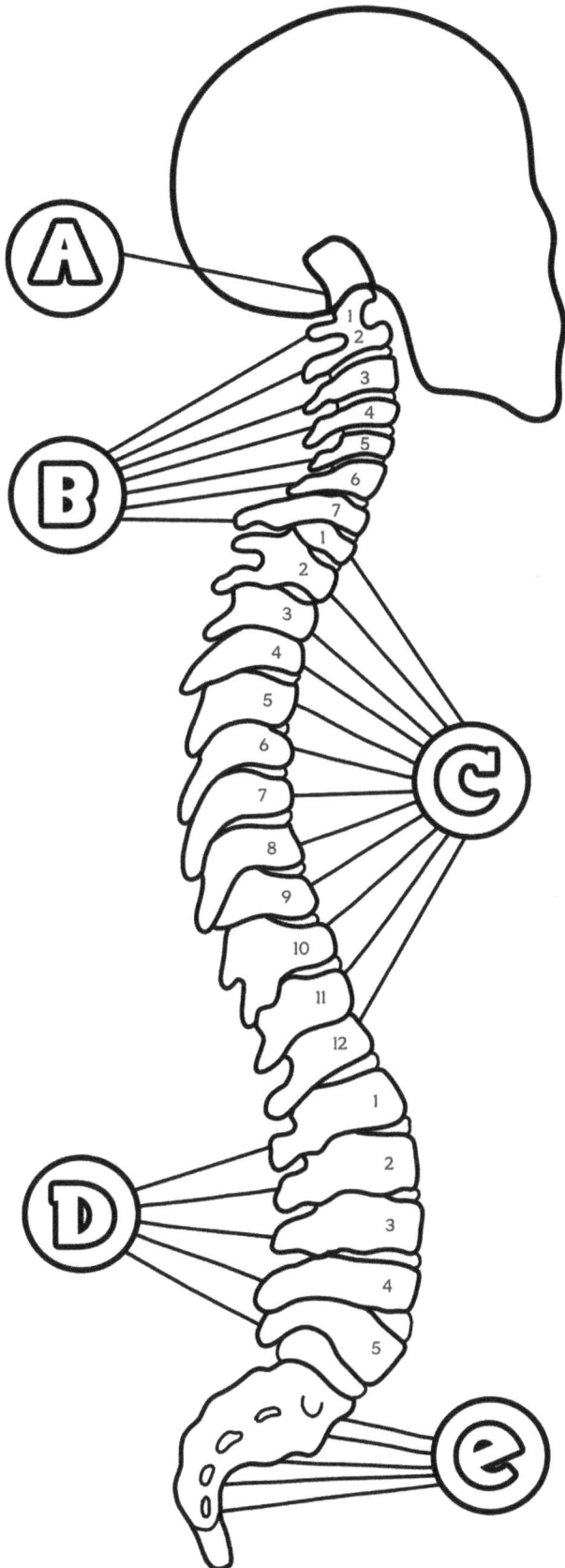

A. CRANIAL NERVES VIA BRAIN STEM

B. CERVICAL NERVES VIA C1-C7

C. THORACIC NERVES VIA T1-T12

D. LUMBAR NERVES VIA L1-L5

E. SACRAL NERVES VIA S1-S5

MVN: Most Valuable Nerve

I know I shouldn't play favorites, but the vagus nerve has superpowers! Being the 10th cranial nerve, it is referred to as 'Cranial Nerve X'...fancy roman numerals for fancy nerves!

When I say superpowers, I mean it does *so many things*! The longest nerve in the body, it starts in your brain and travels all the way down to your colon (with many branches along the way). Vagus actually translates to 'wandering' in Latin. In some ways it's The Boss, because it is responsible for 80-90% of the communication *to the brain* about how things are going in your organs.[14] In the past, we have focused on the messages going in the other direction—from the CNS outwards—but communication is a two-way street, after all! The vagus nerve is like the best babysitter...or maybe a tattletale (you choose), but those constant messages keep you alive! We need a lot of things from our brain, and this nerve tells it what's up.

We touched on the parasympathetic nervous system awhile back, and the vagus nerve is its main squeeze! It is involved in or responsible for a wide array of things such as: involuntary movements like our heart rate, lungs and digestive tract, sweating, speech and gag-reflex/vomiting.

Intense emotional stress can cause the vagus nerve to reduce **cardiac output**, and also cause temporary loss of bladder control. The vagus nerve is greatly implicated in the effects of traumatic brain injury from concussions, including the PTSD suffered by many veterans and injuries to athletes. There are also studies being done stimulating the vagus nerve as a treatment for epilepsy, depression, tinnitus and obesity. The field of **neurogastroenterology** (say that 10 times fast!) is also studying how chronic inflammation in the gut might be negatively affecting the conduction of this nerve, leading to these conditions and more. This field of study explores the intersection of the enteric nervous system and, in part, the role of the vagus nerve in communication.

You can actually stimulate your vagus nerve by singing, humming, deep breathing exercises, laughing, or splashing your face (or body) with cold water...

Now why would you want to do that?!

The vagus nerve is top dog of your parasympathetic nervous system, or the 'rest and digest' one. It regulates your chill mode. The more you stimulate it, the more opportunities your body has to shift out of 'fight/flight/freeze' mode and into a more calm, sustainable state of being.[15]

As boring as breathing sounds, we should do it *WAY* more.

We can see from our coloring sheet that this all-important nerve is all around town... and the function of all of those things is keeping us alive, no joke. When we start seeing the interweaving between physical and emotional health, there really is no separating them. Supporting or healing one has a direct impact on the other.

Interestingly, the vagus nerve is specifically tied to the *exhale*. "During the inhalation phase of a breathing cycle, the sympathetic nervous system facilitates a brief acceleration of heart rate; during exhalation, the vagus nerve secretes a transmitter substance (ACh) which causes deceleration within beat-to-beat intervals via the parasympathetic nervous system" writes Christopher Bergland for Psychology Today.

"One gadget-free way to track the timing of your inhalation-to-exhalation breathing cycles per minute is to use a 4:8 ratio of four-second inhalations and eight-second exhalations."[16]

Let's be honest, inhaling for 4 and exhaling for 8 can be hard! Try 6 and 6, then 4 and 6... one day you will be all 4:8 and feelin' great!

Take yourself down a few notches...your vagus nerve will purr in gratitude!

✴ THE VAGUS NERVE ✴

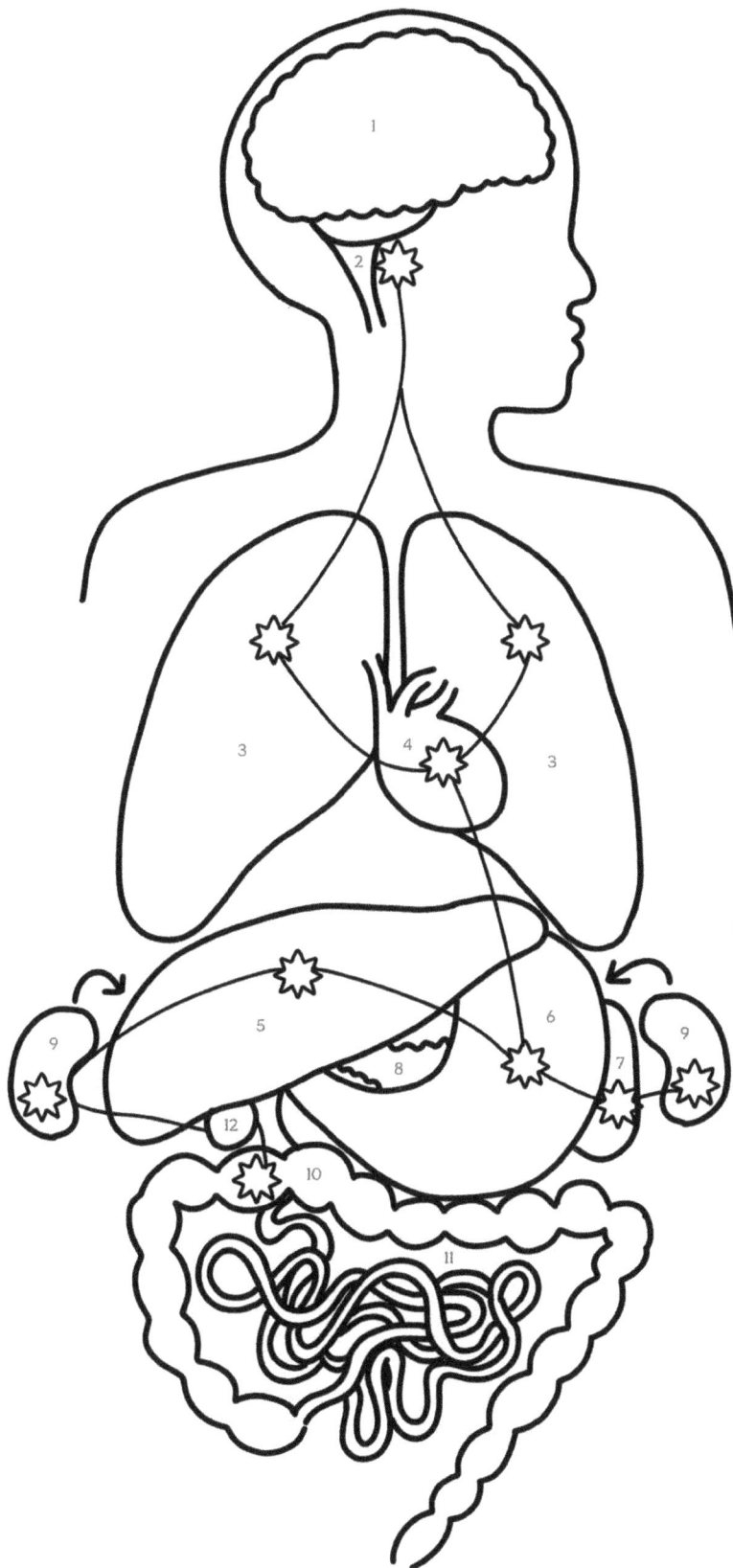

1. BRAIN
2. BRAIN STEM
3. LUNGS
4. HEART
5. LIVER
6. STOMACH
7. SPLEEN
8. PANCREAS
9. KIDNEYS
10. LARGE INTESTINE
11. SMALL INTESTINE
12. GALL BLADDER

The Endocrine System

The world of hormones. Their involvement in your body's function is referred to as the endocrine system. Specifically, **glands** are the structures that secrete hormones. Hormones are chemical messengers, and hormone balancing is a full-time job! If they had a house party, it would be rockin'! There are a ton of different hormones in the body, and their jobs overlap.

Here are the major glands of the endocrine system:

- **Hypothalamus:** Located in the center of the brain, this gland is responsible for overall homeostasis, or balance, of the body's systems. It works with both the endocrine and the nervous systems to do this. Remember the vagus nerve? That is one way the body tells the brain what's up, by sending signals to the hypothalamus. It is responsible for triggering the pituitary to release many of its hormones and supporting many body functions. Using a hormone called GnRh, the hypothalamus stimulates the pituitary to release some of the hormones involved in reproductive function.

- **Pituitary:** Located just below the hypothalamus and oftentimes signaled by it. The pituitary releases many hormones, some of them stimulating *other* glands to release *their* hormones...it's kind of like an intricate relay race!

- **Pineal:** Located in the brain, just behind those folks up there. Some of its function is unknown, but it is involved in melatonin production, which regulates circadian rhythms, the sleep patterns you have in response to darkness or light. Side note: Screen time at night messes with it! Your eyes are not good at filtering out this kind of light, so it goes right into your retina, and actually *blocks* the melatonin, making you less sleepy.[17] All types of computers emit this blue light, but so do TV, fluorescent and LED lights. Cutting yourself off from the gadgets and turning down the lights a couple of hours before bed can be an 'easy' fix for restless nights. I know, it's hard...but that social media post will be there tomorrow! And you'll be really cool if you're like, "whatever, I was busy."

- **Thyroid:** This gland influences metabolism, growth rate and body temperature by releasing various thyroid hormones. It can be dysregulated by stress.

- **Parathyroid:** Regulates calcium levels in the blood and bones. We use calcium for the function of many organ systems, so it has its own gland to keep it in check.

- **Thymus:** The thymus produces and grows t-cells, which are a main component of your immune system. T-cells destroy pathogens and cancer cells. T-cells like to hang out in your lymph nodes, waiting for the lymphatic fluid to bring them stuff to destroy!

- **Pancreas:** The pancreas is both an organ and a gland! The main hormones it releases are insulin (to lower blood sugar), and glucagon (to raise blood sugar). Blood sugar balance affects *everything*, as you might know from your hangrier moments. The pancreas also releases **digestive enzymes**, to help you break down your food into its many usable parts.

- **Adrenals:** Situated on top of each kidney, the adrenal glands secrete adrenaline and steroid hormones. These hormones help regulate blood pressure and are involved in your stress-response. They also help with metabolism, immune response and other body functions.

- **Ovaries:** In addition to growing eggs, the ovaries secrete hormones, mainly estrogen and progesterone, which are main players in reproductive function and overall health.

- **Testes:** In addition to growing sperm, the testes secrete testosterone, which is a main player in reproductive function and overall health.

THE ENDOCRINE SYSTEM

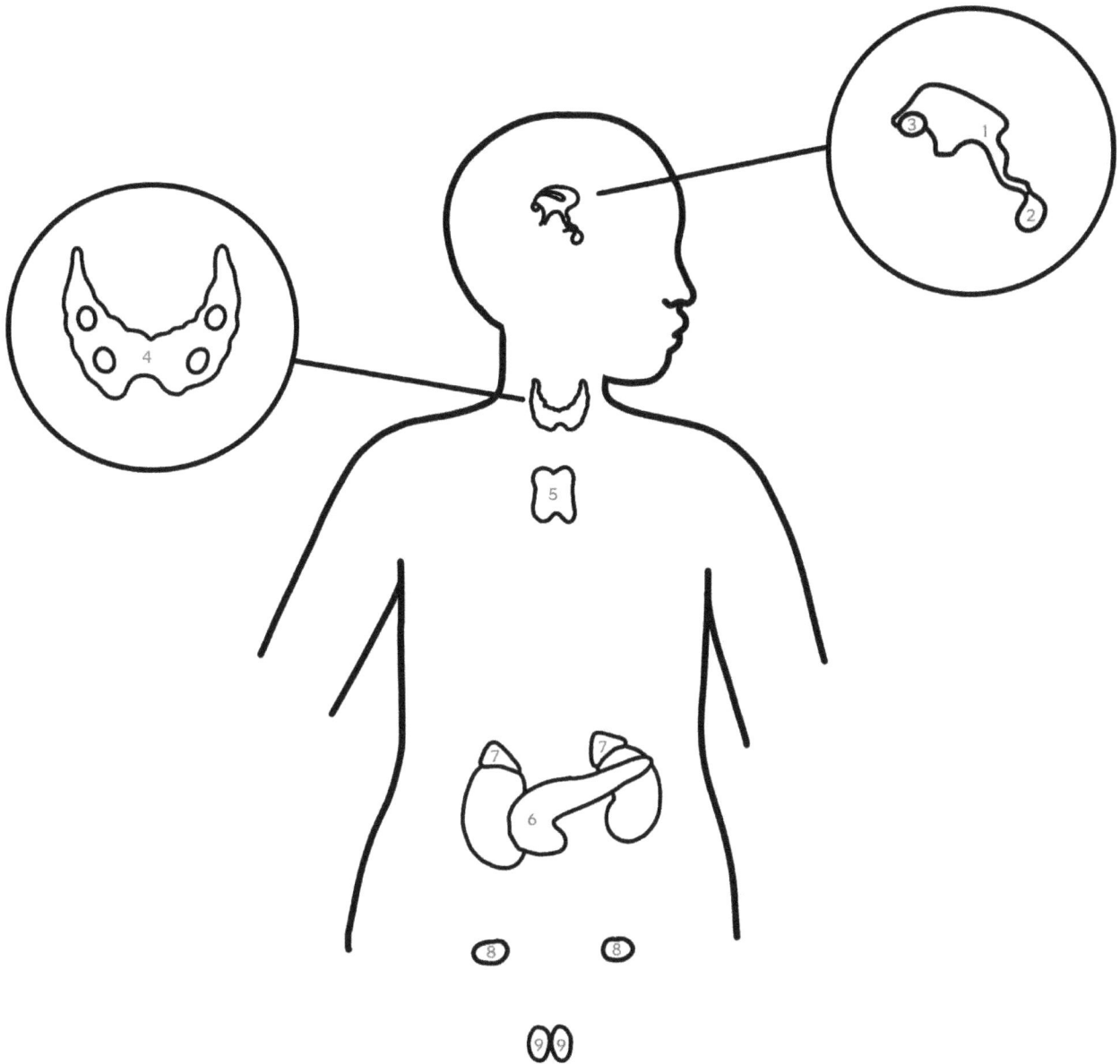

1. HYPOTHALAMUS
2. PITUITARY 3. PINEAL
4. THYROID/PARATHYROID
5. THYMUS 6. PANCREAS
7. ADRENALS
8. OVARIES 9. TESTES

So Many Hormones,
So Little Time...

There are around 50 hormones circulating in the human body. Here are some of the most popular ones and a glance at their roles. They exist in varying levels based on time of day, time of month, life stage, health, stage of digestion/elimination, biological sex, hormonal interventions and individual makeup!

Just for fun, I've also included a couple of neurotransmitters (dopamine and endorphins). Neurotransmitters are chemical messengers that function within the nervous system, whereas hormones are chemicals of the endocrine system — but they work together sometimes![18]

- **GnRH (Gonadotropin releasing hormone):** Released by the hypothalamus. Stimulates the pituitary to release LH and FSH.

- **LH (Luteinizing hormone):** Released by the pituitary. Stimulates ovulation and production of testosterone.

- **FSH (Follicle-stimulating hormone):** Released by the pituitary. Stimulates follicle maturation and sperm production by triggering the ovaries and testes, respectively.

- **Estrogen:** Three types, produced by the ovaries, placenta and testes. Stimulates sex development during puberty, endometrial and uterine growth, blood vessel and skin maintenance, decreases bone *resorption*, increases creation of protein-binding cells in the liver, sodium and water retention, reduces bowel motility, supports alveoli in the lungs, and more!

- **Progesterone:** Released in the ovaries, adrenal glands, and placenta. Supports fertility, pregnancy and birth. Also a muscle relaxer, immune regulator, assists thyroid function, bone, skin, teeth, gums, joint, tendon and ligament health, nerve function, cancer prevention (by balancing estrogen), and more!

- **Testosterone:** Released by the testes and ovaries. In a group of steroid hormones called androgens, testosterone is involved in sex drive, sex development during puberty, muscle mass, bone density, and is a key ingredient to sperm production. As with all other hormones, healthy levels affect many aspects of overall health.

- **Prostaglandin:** Mitigates injury and illness by controlling inflammation, blood flow and clotting; also involved in the induction of labor.

- **Oxytocin:** The "bonding hormone." Released by the pituitary. Stimulates release of breast milk. Stimulates contraction of cervix and vagina (whether during sex or childbirth). Involved in orgasm, ejaculation, breastfeeding, trust and connection between people and other sentient beings, body temperature, wakefulness.

- **Thyroid hormones:** Released by the pituitary and thyroid. Regulates body temperature, metabolism and heart rate.

- **Insulin:** Produced by the pancreas. Regulates blood sugar.

- **Ghrelin and leptin:** Released by the stomach. Stimulate appetite and satiety (fullness), respectively.

- **Prolactin:** Released by the pituitary and stimulates breast growth and lactation.

- **Serotonin:** Key hormone that stimulates our feelings of well-being; found in the brain, bowels and blood platelets. Inflammation in the gut can impair its ability to function.

- **Cortisol:** A main component of the stress-response. Most body cells have cortisol receptors, so it has many functions: blood sugar, salt/water balance and blood pressure are just a few. High levels occur with chronic stress, and dysregulated sleep can have a domino effect on healthy levels.

- **Adrenalin:** Released by the adrenal glands to speed up functions related to physical exertion by increasing circulation, breathing and carbohydrate metabolism.

- **Dopamine:** A neurotransmitter produced in the hypothalamus and other brain structures, dopamine has many functions including boosting your mood, supporting the sympathetic (action-based) nervous system, inhibiting prolactin and increasing your motivation. It also has a role in your motor and cognitive function as well as your decision making and impulse control.

- **Endorphins:** A neurotransmitter produced in the pituitary and the central nervous system, endorphins are released to reduce pain, boost mood and wellbeing. Their release is triggered by pain, stress and activities like exercise, eating and sex, to name a few. They help us feel good, which in turn enhances our quality of life by supporting activities that make us happy...which then produces more endorphins! It's a happy cause-and-effect cycle!

HORMONE HUNT

```
S E N D O R P H I N S F P N O
P O B C P H R C P e Q O A F M
R T H Y R O i D F S H L D D T
O S S P O P A P i e F L R H B
G A T i S i S R N R N i e O N
e i D T B C i S O R C N R i
S S M M A H O T U T U L A M Q
T T U P G C R A L O B e L O L
e R L C L U T e i N i Z i N G
R O A S A R i D N i O A N e S
O G T B N i S C P N X H e C P
N e i G D N O S D C Y D K Y R
e N N F i T L L e P T i N T O
H B G O N A D O T R O P i N L
i D O P A M i N e T C K R P A
L T R P R e L e A S i N G e C
D S G H R e L i N W N F M H T
V D S G N R H P O L V D T P i
K O T e S T O S T e R O N e N
i P F J A G U U P R U i J B A
```

ADRENALINE

CORTISOL

DOPAMINE

ENDORPHINS

ESTROGEN

FOLLICLE

FSH

GHRELIN

GNRH

GONADOTROPIN

HORMONE

INSULIN

LEPTIN

LH

LUTEINIZING

OXYTOCIN

PROGESTERONE

PROLACTIN

PROSTAGLANDIN

RELEASING

SEROTONIN

STIMULATING

TESTOSTERONE

THYROID

Introducing... Your Uterus!

Well, okay... maybe you have one, **maybe you don't.** But they are *amazing*! To be fair, all organs are pretty rad, but this one does some fabulous tricks in perfectly choreographed fashion. And I'm fairly certain you came out of one!

This system is perfectly designed to prepare eggs ready for fertilization, to transport an egg to the place where it can connect with sperm (should any be hanging around), to create an environment supportive of embryo development, to grow an entire human life, and, when there is no pregnancy, to shed an internal layer so as to be ready for another cycle. Whew! The communication between the brain, ovaries and uterus is dynamic!

Here are the parts that make up the whole of it:

- **Os:** The opening to the uterus. To prevent bacteria from entering, the os is closed unless menstrual flow, cervical mucus, a baby or sperm are passing through. Hormonal triggers tell the os what to do when...as with everything else!

- **Cervix:** The very base of the uterus. Nestled into the top of the vaginal canal, this structure needs to both be strong enough to help keep a growing fetus in, but also to soften and open during birth. It also provides some of the 'scaffolding' that supports surrounding structures, such as the bladder. A complete hysterectomy would remove the cervix, but if there is not a specific reason to do so, leaving it can help to maintain bladder and pelvic strength. During the birthing process, the cervix needs to open to a certain diameter for baby to pass through, and sometimes stress or emotional tension can prevent that![19] It is a great example of how emotions can have a direct effect on our physical function.

- **Neck and body:** Forming the center of the uterus, this section is very muscular and vascular (containing a network of blood vessels), which helps with the contractions necessary during both menstruation and childbirth.

- **Fundus:** Top portion of the uterus. Ideally peaks just above the level of the pubic bone, behind the bladder. Also very muscular and vascular, this section is the most mobile as the uterus changes size during a menstrual cycle or a pregnancy. The networks of blood vessels in the uterus need to not only support the organ itself, but also sustain a baby (via the *placenta*).

- **Vagina** (or vaginal canal): Starting just after the labia minora, this passage leads up to the base of the uterus, or cervix. People often refer to the *external* genitalia as the vagina, but in reality, what we see on the outside is the labia majora and mons pubis, the labia minora, the clitoris and a number of other structures, all of which are called the vulva.

- **Ovaries**: At birth, the ovaries contain ALL of the eggs you have for your lifetime! Fun fact: ovaries are fully formed when a baby is developing in the uterus, at about 4.5 months gestational age. At that time, the ovaries hold around 6-7 million eggs. By the time the baby is born, there are just 1-2 million remaining, and by the time puberty hits, there are around 300,000 left to last a lifetime! So, if you are carrying a baby with ovaries beyond the 4.5-month point, the eggs that might eventually become your grandchildren (should they want them or have them) are inside you too! Multi-generational housing, to say the least! Also quite beautiful, if you're the poetic type.

- **Fallopian tubes:** The passage the egg travels through from the fimbriae to the uterus. This is most commonly where fertilization occurs, as the sperm have usually made their way to the egg in one of these tubes. An ectopic pregnancy is when the fertilized egg implants inside the tube instead of traveling down into the uterus, which can be dangerous and does not support a full-term pregnancy. The fallopian tubes are what are cut and tied in a tubal ligation, a permanent birth control option.

- **Fimbriae:** Fingerlike projections that scoop up the ovulated egg into the fallopian tube. PS — they don't really look like flames — that's me taking creative license...go with it, people!

- **Endometrium** (or endometrial lining): The innermost layer of the uterus that provides a surface for implantation of a fertilized embryo. This lining thickens, filling with the nutrients necessary to support a growing embryo during the menstrual cycle, or sheds when no pregnancy occurs during menstruation.

THE UTERUS + FRIENDS

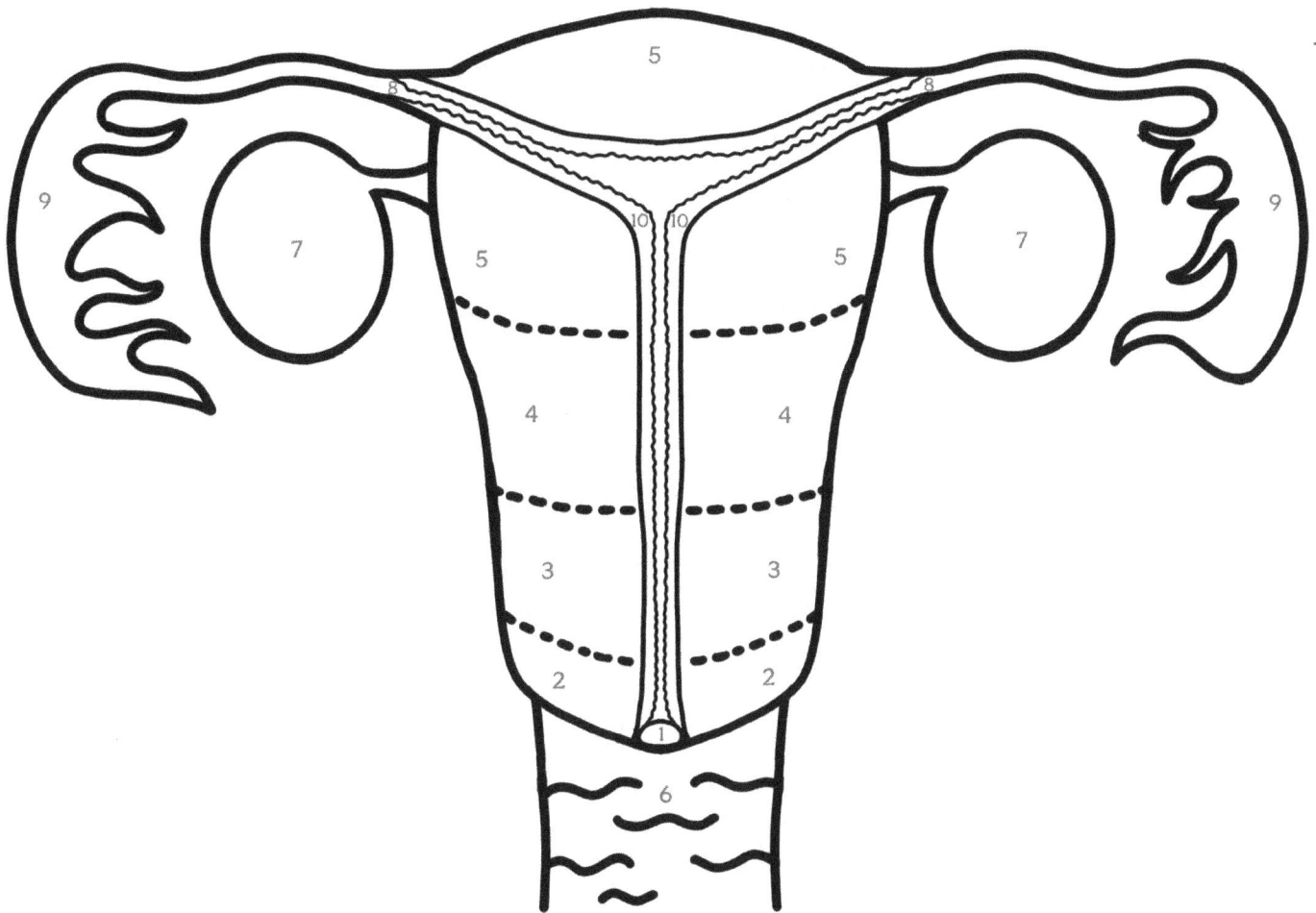

1. OS
2. CERVIX
3. NECK
4. BODY
5. FUNDUS

6. VAGINA
7. OVARY
8. FALLOPIAN TUBE
9. FIMBRIAE
10. ENDOMETRIUM

Ligaments for Days...

These are all of the ligaments that keep the uterus and its related structures positioned properly for any kind of action.[20]

Crazy, right?! Uterine and ovarian ligaments are designed to act as supportive guides that help to maintain the *integrity of the position* and *orientation* of the womb. Very important events occur within these structures, and their positioning is related to the function of them! Remember when I said that ligaments go from bone-to-bone? I sort of lied. Ligaments attached to organs do their own thing, often interweaving with the surrounding tissue...which *eventually* leads to a bone.

The uterus is surrounded by other organs and is the most mobile organ in the body! While the lower portion (the neck and cervix) are nestled into place, the middle and upper portion need to have the space to double in size during a menstrual cycle, and *many times* in size during the course of a pregnancy...so it needs to be free!

Why are there so many ligaments if it needs to be free, you ask? The ligaments serve to encourage optimal placement...guidance, not restriction! We need everything to be oriented ideally for the egg to be released and scooped up by the fimbriae, and to travel down the tiny fallopian tube. We also need the uterus's contractions to be strong enough to effectively expel its lining each month during menstruation, and also to expel the babe during birth. Very important things, right?

Just like muscles pulling on bones, too much tension on a ligament over time creates a problem. Various factors can cause some of the uterine ligaments to be too tight. Surgery, for example, can create scar tissue. If the scar tissue isn't addressed (with scar massage), it can start to spread and cause restriction in surrounding tissues. Injury is another common cause of uterine binding. If you injure your hip and those muscles are tight for an extended period of time, the fascia surrounding them can pull the uterus towards them and hold it in an off-center place. 'Hold it' is the issue in question here... we want the uterus to be free to move.

What is fascia, anyways?

Fascia is a very strong (yet thin) tissue that surrounds all of our muscles and organs. It is interconnected throughout the body, so tension in one area pulls on other areas. Tight fascia surrounding the muscles on the inside of your hip can easily pull on the fascia of nearby structures, such as the uterus. A sedentary lifestyle, often a job requirement, also creates tight fascia in the pelvis, simply from so many hours spent with little to no movement and circulation. Like muscles, fascia wants to move!

So take that womb for a walk! It's important to keep the uterus moving, along with the rest of the body! Gentle yoga, walking, avoiding a sedentary lifestyle, bodywork (including abdominal/uterine massage if indicated by menstrual difficulties, pathologies or fertility issues), proper nutrition, plenty of water, and avoiding toxins will...

FREE THE UTERUS!

Some of the same stretches indicated for the psoas muscle are great for the uterus: Warrior, Pigeon, Child's, Reclining Bound Angle poses are all great yoga positions. There are whole sequences for the hips, menstruation, fertility...you name it, there are yoga poses for it! Remember, overstretching is very common in yoga, so go to the beginning of the stretch sensation and hold. Learn how to use props to support you in that spot. A little bit of stretch goes a long way!

When the uterus is *twice* it's normal size and weight, before and during menstruation, those ligaments are extra sensitive to strain—like heavy lifting, running (especially on hard surfaces) or hard labor of any kind. Your body is trying to do this big thing, so if you can take it a bit easy during the week leading up to and during menses, those ligaments will thank you for not having to double-time it. This does not mean that you shouldn't move or get exercise...movement can be good! Just take it down to the gentler side of life for a spell.

LIGAMENTS!

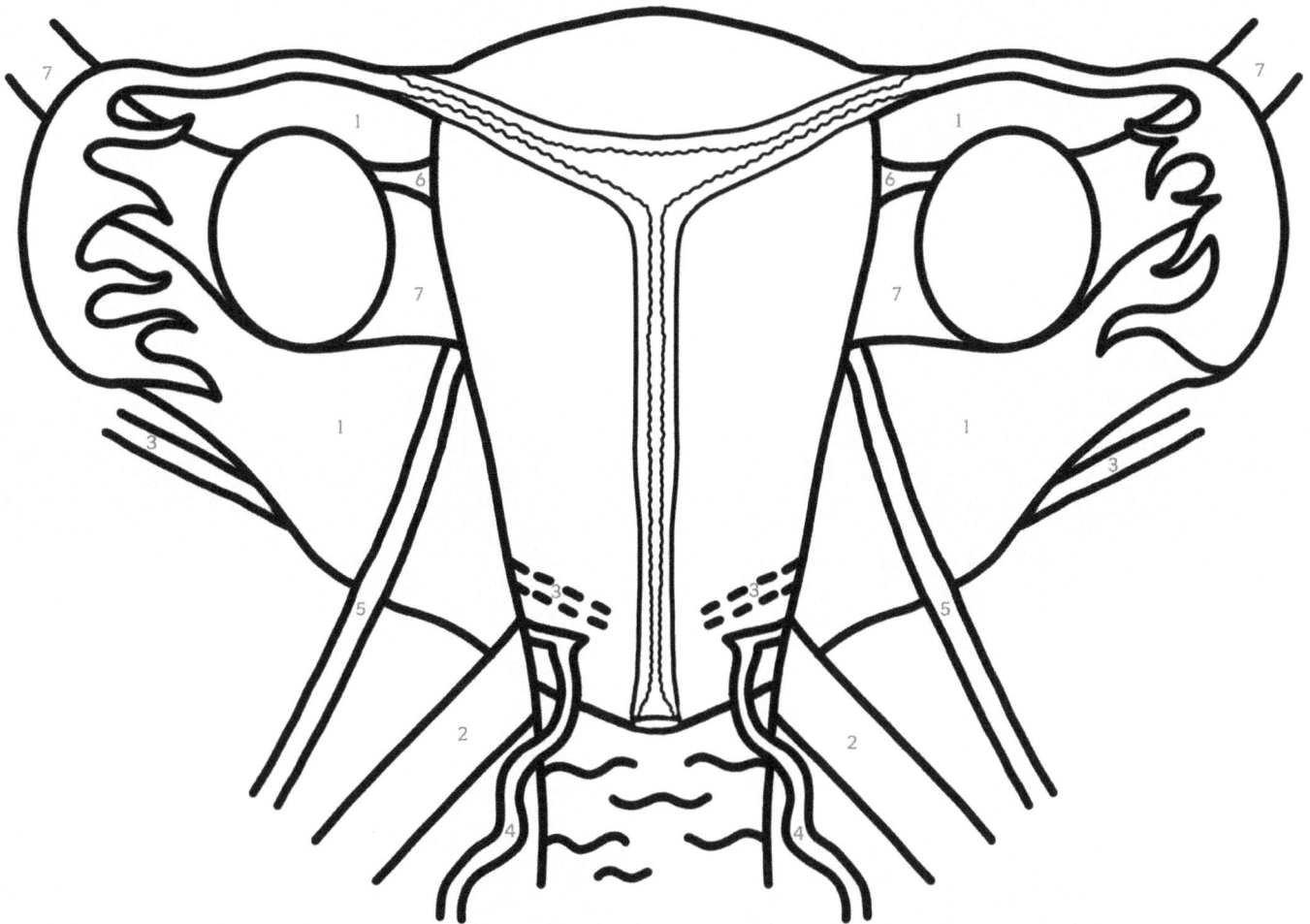

UTERINE:
1. BROAD
2. CARDINAL
3. UTERO-SACRAL
4. PUBO-CERVICAL
5. ROUND

OVARIAN:
6. PROPER
7. SUSPENSORY

Where *Is* That Womb?

You might have noticed by now that I'm using the word, "womb." It's not a word I used to feel drawn to, but I have come to appreciate that it encompasses both the whole physical structure, and the energetic space therein. 'Uterus' leaves out the ovaries and fallopian tubes, and can sound pretty clinical. I also want to convey that there is an energetic space in the pelvis to develop a relationship with, regardless of life events (such as a partial or complete **hysterectomy**) or your **sex assigned at birth** (based on your external anatomy). I say this partially because some people develop a disdain for their bodies, either due to societal messages, physical pain, **gender dysphoria**, or **body dysmorphia**. That kind of stress can have a real-life impact on pelvic health! Whatever the future holds for you and your body, it is surely doing the best it can, and it deserves props! Whatever you've got in your pelvis, try to be kind to it!

In *The Body Is Not An Apology*, Sonya Renee Taylor points out that, "We did not start life in a negative partnership with our bodies. I have never seen a toddler lament the size of their thighs, the squishiness of their belly. Children do not arrive here ashamed of their race, gender, age or differing abilities. Babies LOVE their bodies! Each discovery they encounter is freaking awesome! Have you ever seen an infant realize they have feet? Talk about wonder." She goes on, "You must make peace with your body.... You did not come to the planet hating your body. What if you accepted the fact that much of how you view your body and your judgments of it are *learned* things, messages you have deeply internalized that have created an adversarial relationship. Hating your body is like finding a person you despise and then choosing to spend the rest of your life with them while loathing every moment of the partnership."[21]

Not hating our bodies in this culture can be hard, but remember what that baby would say and how much they would love you, regardless of anything. Be that baby, for yourself and for others.

So, back to the womb and where you might find it. Many people mistakenly think it's located in the lower abdomen...but it's really housed by the pelvis. Here we have the general order of things: pubic bone > bladder > uterus > bowel > sacrum. Of course, these structures are not suspended in the body like some sort of organ circus... they are surrounded by fascia, muscles, the circulatory and nervous system, the lymphatic system, and other organs. It's cozy in there!

In the next pages, we will go over some less-than-ideal circumstances for the womb to be in. I don't want to scare you, but understanding the function (and dysfunction) of our bodies can really help us catch and address issues sooner-than-later going forward. Let's set you up for success!

We don't always know what causes some of these conditions, but we can make some educated guesses at factors that play a role:

- **Stress**, as evidenced by studies done on how elevated cortisol levels affect physical health.[22] Stress can prevent ovulation, increase muscle tension which decreases blood flow, and affect hormone and neurotransmitter levels which affects everything!

- **Environment**, as evidenced by areas with high incidence rates.[23] This can be a difficult one to control, outside of changing your location, successful environmental activism and access to clean water, air and healthy food. There are also health disparities faced by marginalized and oppressed groups when societies remain ignorant and blind to their treatment of these individuals and families. Uncovering overt and unconscious bias in our systems and enacting policy changes should be built into all just and equitable societies.

- **Diet/lifestyle** as evidenced by the effectiveness of changes in diet and lifestyle on improving dis-ease conditions.[24] Related to environmental concerns, your body thrives well on whole foods. Tons of vegetables, some quality protein, and fruits and grains. We know this. But people are making mad profit off of our addiction to junk! Try adding in good things instead of taking things away. Changing one habit at a time is more sustainable than going cold turkey on everything you love and then crashing off the wagon!

- **Genetics**, as evidenced by...genetics. It is actually difficult to study the genetic connections separate from the environmental ones.[25] Knowing your family medical history is very important if possible... but don't use it as your own rap sheet... *you* are *you*, not them!

- **Accident, injury, surgery,** as evidenced by the effects of scar tissue and fascial restrictions.[26] We talked about this earlier. Scar tissue is very important for healing a wound, so don't condemn it... but over time it starts trying to take up more and more real estate, and that can cause restriction or tension.

Where there's a womb, there's a way... that's what I say!

WHERE IS THAT WOMB?

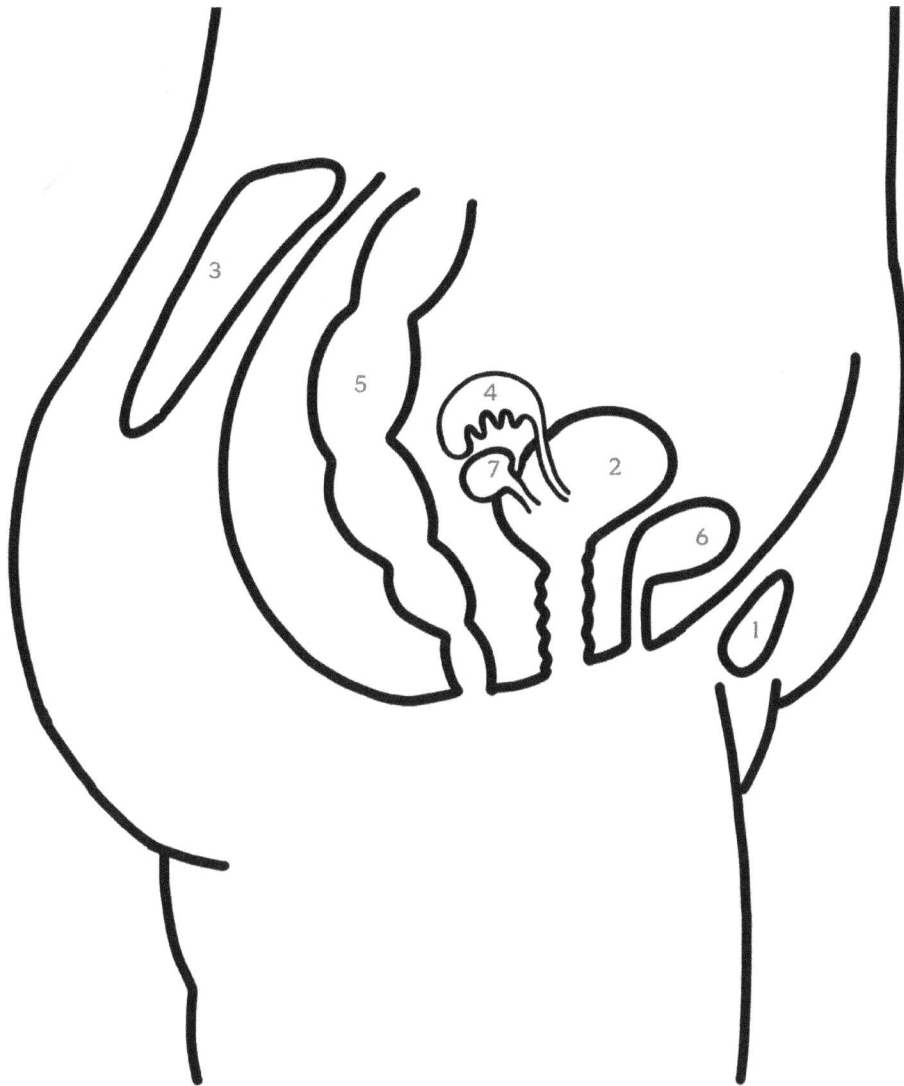

1. PUBIC BONE
2. UTERUS
3. SACRUM
4. FALLOPIAN TUBE/FIMBRAE
5. BOWEL
6. BLADDER
7. OVARY

Stuck on You...

Remember when I said that the uterus is the most mobile organ in the body? It's true! But sometimes it gets off center and stuck there! Beyond a specific event (such as an injury or surgery), this can be caused over time or exacerbated by the things we've talked about: sedentary living, heavy lifting just before and during menses, running frequently on hard surfaces, a difficult childbirth or just the muscle laxity that happens with age.[27]

Here are some positions your uterus might find itself in:

- **Retroversion:** Uterus stuck back towards the rectum. Symptoms can be low back pain and/or dark stool before menses, hemorrhoids, and significant menstrual cramps. Dark and clotty blood during menses. Because the uterus is restricted near the rectum, it can have an effect on your bowel movements, causing constipation and sometimes also diarrhea.

- **Retroflexion:** Uterus folded over and stuck backwards towards the rectum. Similar symptoms to retroversion, but more extreme. The uterus will have a harder time evacuating the endometrial lining during menses, and this can also have an effect on fertility.

- **Anteversion:** Uterus stuck forward towards the bladder. Can result in urinary issues and/or increase in urinary tract infections. It's no fun to have something pressing on your bladder! When the uterus is causing restriction in this area, you might have a hard time holding your pee, urinate frequently or, depending on where the restriction is, have a difficult time getting your pee out.

- **Anteflexion:** Uterus folded over and stuck forward towards the bladder. Similar symptoms to anteversion, but more extreme. Again, this is going to make the tasks of the uterus more difficult.

- **Uterine prolapse:** Uterus descends into the vaginal canal. Classified in 1st-4th degree depending on severity. You can also have a prolapse of the bladder (cystocele) or the rectum (rectocele), which means that the wall between those organs and the vaginal canal is injured, and that organ pushes towards or into the vaginal canal. Symptoms can include urinary or bowel issues, heaviness in the pelvis, feeling pressure or tissue change in the vaginal canal. Most often happens after a difficult childbirth or as an elder due to natural tissue changes coupled with life events.

- **Tilt (left or right):** Uterus stuck to one side or another. Symptoms can include hip pain on that side, especially leading up to menses, failure to ovulate or painful ovulation. This can affect the positioning of the ovary and fallopian tubes and their function, and/or overstretch the ligaments on the other side, possibly causing pain to that hip.

Uterine position is a large part of what my teacher's teacher (Don Elijio Panti) focused on in his rural jungle medical practice in Belize. An indigenous healer of physical, emotional and spiritual illnesses, he was renowned in Central America for healing even the most difficult of conditions. Traditional medicine was more integrated than our modern version of healthcare. You didn't go to a different doctor for every different body part and/or emotional struggle...it was believed to be all connected! A uterus that was 'off-center' (or stuck) put the whole person off center, body and mind. In addition to abdominal massage to loosen and restore blood, lymphatic and nervous flow, the energetic and spiritual self needed to flow as well! In his tradition, that might mean the burning of copal incense with prayers and a spiritual bath with the beautiful flowers of the region.

This might sound new and different to you, but some form of these practices existed (and still do!) in all indigenous cultures of the world. We are remembering, bit-by-bit, that these old ways actually do work, and transformation can, in certain circumstances, be impossible without them! There are traditional healers worldwide that have carried these practices forward through the generations and are great resources to our communities!

It can be fun to look up the folk healing practices, plants and traditions of your own ancestry. Learn about the wisdom of your past and how people are using it today!

VARIATIONS ON UTERINE POSITION

RETRO-VERSION

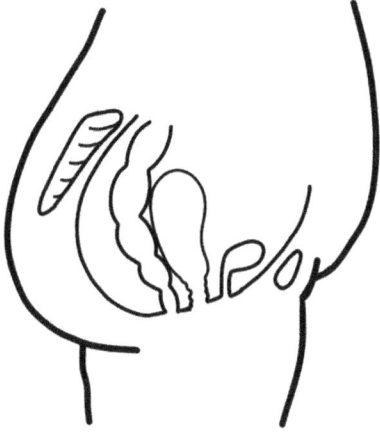

RETRO-FLEXION

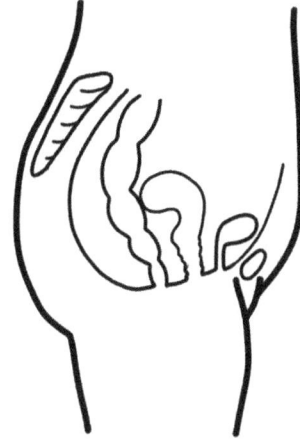

ANTE-VERSION

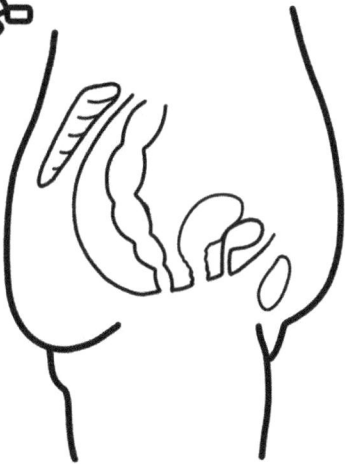

ANTE-FLEXION

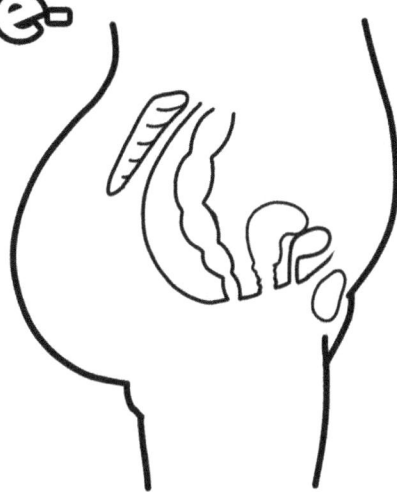

LATERAL TILT

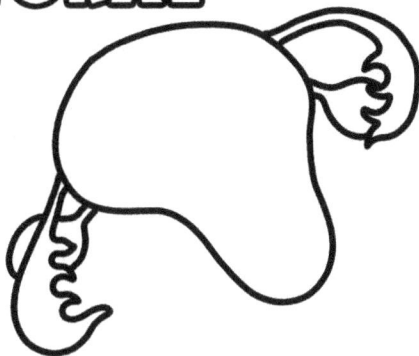

UTERINE PROLAPSE

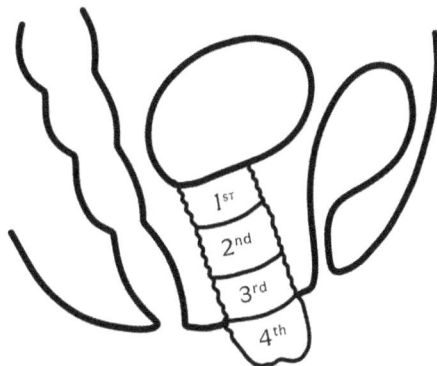

1st
2nd
3rd
4th

SOS to the Uterus!

This image illustrates the most common *pathologies* that can happen to the uterus and ovaries...in one womb! *All* of these imbalances in one body would never happen in actual life...it's a dramatized version of a womb in distress! If you end up with one of these conditions it can be a difficult time, but you are not necessarily destined to misery and pain. There are ***holistic*** and ***allopathic*** answers galore! Research, make lists of questions, and find trusted practitioners to work with. It will likely take trial-and-error, but you are resourceful! Here is a list of the ailments illustrated, all laid out in their pathological glory:

- **Endometriosis/adenomyosis:** These two conditions involve the endometrial layer of the uterus (remember that one?). With endometriosis, endometrial cells end up *outside* the uterus. Those cells, wherever they end up, continue to behave like they do on the inside, meaning they react to your reproductive hormones by getting inflamed and bleeding during menstruation. They can end up anywhere, but are most often found around the uterus, lower bowel and inside the pelvis. The inflammation can also cause ***adhesions*** and ***scar tissue*** to form, which can restrict the function of muscles or organs.

It is also not-so-pleasant to have tiny menstrual cycles happening in multiple places inside your body! The severity of endometriosis varies greatly from person to person. Adenomyosis occurs inside the uterus but acts the same way, with endometrial cells infiltrating the other layers of the uterus.

- **Fibroids:** Also called fibroid tumors, fibroids are solid masses, usually inside the uterus but not always. They are notably dense, or hard, compared with other pathologies. Fibroids themselves are not *necessarily* a problem, but they are a sign of imbalance, and can cause excessive menstrual bleeding, obstruct bladder or bowel function, or be in the way of optimal implantation of a fertilized egg. The size of fibroids varies greatly.

This is one of the issues that shows up in racial health disparities in the US: African Americans are more likely to develop fibroids, to develop them earlier, and to have surgeries and ongoing difficulties related to them. The reasons for this are many and sobering. The stress of navigating a racist society (stress = stress hormones, which can = ill-health) and the racist way Black people are treated in the medical system are two causes.[28]

Racial disparities also affect other people of color and health disparities exist in all marginalized/oppressed groups. This is a call-to-action for our citizens and leaders to change the systemic health disparities across racial and economic groups!

- **Polyps**: These are an overgrowth of cells out of the endometrial lining of the uterus (but attached to it). They are most often non-cancerous (but not always), and you can have one or many. Polyps can also form in the colon, which is why a colonoscopy is recommended later in life to ensure there is no cancer growth.

- **Polycystic ovarian syndrome (PCOS)**: PCOS is a condition where many follicles develop on the ovaries, but they fail to ovulate, and don't dissipate throughout the cycle. Menstrual irregularity and excess androgen hormones are often associated with this condition, and 40% of people with PCOS develop prediabetes. Changes in diet/lifestyle are a main treatment, as it is connected to blood sugar levels and hormone dysregulation. There are both natural and pharmaceutical recommendations, as well. Take time to research and see what your body responds to—and, as always, pay attention to potential side effects of all remedies.

- **Cysts**: Cysts *can* be cancerous, but aren't always. In fact, it's normal for small cysts to grow on your ovaries during ovulation and then dissipate afterwards. Cancer can develop on the ovaries, inside the uterine lining, on the cervix, in the colon...really, anywhere in the body.

Regular pelvic exams and communication with medical practitioners when you are experiencing changes or symptoms is very important for early detection. Please be mindful of anything new or different in your cycle or your abdominal, pelvic or breast tissue.

- **Scar tissue:** Scar tissue can form in and/or around the uterus from various root causes. A widespread infection from an STI or *Asherman's syndrome* are two potential causes. A general term used to describe the results of these conditions (and the pain and discomfort of them) is pelvic inflammatory disease (PID). It can take time and effort to get to the root of PID and often requires a multifaceted approach.

- **Honorable mention:** If you have breasts, take the time to do a self-breast exam at least once a month, just after menstruation if you menstruate. This is the time when breast tissue is the least lumpy and bumpy due to normal hormone fluctuations, so you can feel irregularities and it will be easier to compare with other months if you do it around the same time. If you don't menstruate, put it on the calendar! Forty percent of breast cancers are detected by self-exam — you have the power in your hands!

UTERINE PATHOLOGIES

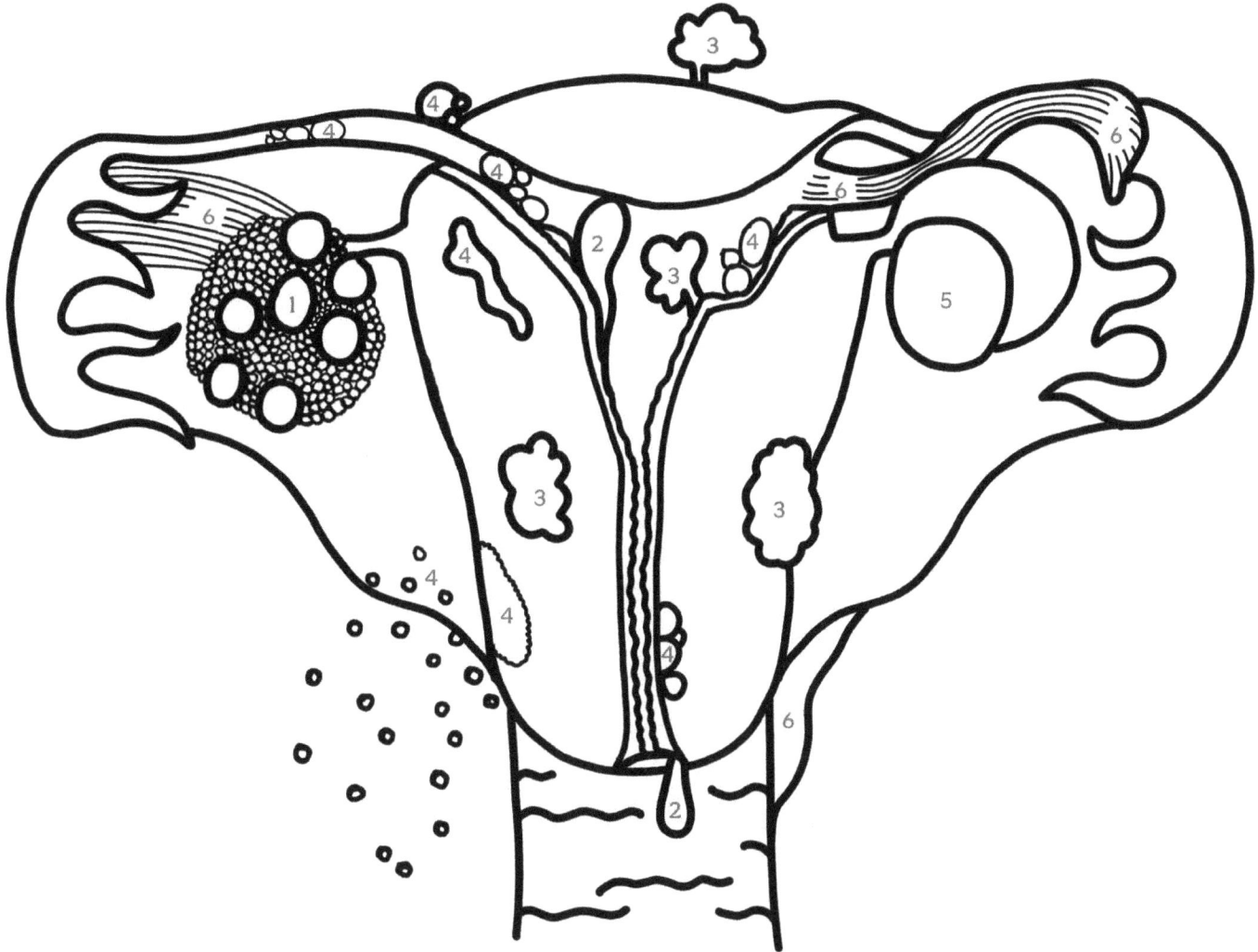

1. PCOS
2. POLYP
3. FIBROID
4. ENDOMETRIOSIS/ADENOMYOSIS
5. OVARIAN CYST
6. ADHESIONS

Introducing . . . Your Prostate!

That's okay if you don't have one, but they rock! This system never gets a break, but it doesn't want one because it's in the sperm-making groove! There really isn't a word like 'womb' for the entirety of this system and its energy, but there *should* be one. I think you should name it something great!

This 24/7 sperm production system is intricately designed to give every one of those millions of sperm the best possible chance at success! Scientists used to believe that there was a 'race' to reach the egg, but that has been disproven.[29] It is an example of humans projecting their own behaviors onto science. All of the conditions are prepared, and the nutrients provided to send these sperm off in tip-top shape (although most of them will perish).

Here are the main components:

- **Ureters:** These two tubes run from the kidneys into the bladder, bringing metabolic waste, filtered out by the kidneys, on the way out as urine.

- **Bladder:** Sometimes called the 'urinary bladder'. We will get into what happens when there is a backup in this system in a bit, but ideally, it's a one-way street!

- **Vas deferens:** This is the tube that transports mature sperm all the way to the urethra. There are some important things that happen along the way, but this is the path. The vas deferens, just above the testes, is what is cut in a vasectomy, an effective birth control option.

- **Prostate gland:** The prostate is generally around the size of a walnut, and it is both muscular and glandular! This means that it contracts (like a muscle) to aid in a speedy ejaculation, but it also produces prostatic fluid to add to the semen. You might notice that the urethra goes *right through* the prostate...crazy, right?! For good reason, semen and urine happen at different moments, so when the prostate contracts, the doorway to the bladder closes...whew, *that's* good news!

- **Testes:** The testes contain a network of tubes called seminal vesicles. The cells inside these tubes react to the testosterone produced by the testes and turn into sperm! The position of the testes (below the pelvis) is designed to regulate their temperature, which is why tight clothing can have an effect on fertility. The scrotum is the pouch that holds the testes. The skin of the scrotum has little folds in it, which makes cleaning and drying it very important!

- **Bulbourethral gland:** We are lucky that these tidy little glands are there to clean out the urethra before the semen comes through. Before ejaculation occurs, these glands release fluid that cleans and kills any bacteria hanging around.

- **Penis:** Well, you've probably heard of them ;-). They come in all shapes, sizes and colors, and following a cascade of psychological and physical events, they can have an erection! The psychological factors can be complex, but a few good ingredients are safety, excitement, and energy. The neural (nerve) factors we talked about earlier with how nerves pass through the central to the peripheral nervous system. The vascular factors are all about blood...blood engorges the penis, making it stiff and erect. And we know some stuff about the endocrine factors...but we will learn more (hint: testosterone!).

- **Seminal vesicles:** These coily little structures produce much of the important components of semen: food for energy, immune support, thickeners...all in a perfectly alkaline form, which help the sperm survive on their journey to the egg!

- **Urethra:** Considered a duct, this tube is the final path of both urine and semen out of the body.

- **Epididymis:** This is where the sperm go to mature and hang out before their big moment. It's like high school...but maybe better!

THE PROSTATE AND FRIENDS

1. URETER (2)
2. BLADDER
3. PROSTATE GLAND

4. SCROTUM
5. PENIS
6. TESTIS (2)

10. URETHRA

11. EPIDIDYMIS (2)

7. VAS DEFERENS (2)
8. BULBOURETHRAL GLAND (2)
9. SEMINAL VESICLE (2)

The Urogenital System

Let's step back and have a look at this system in its entirety. Referred to as the urogenital system, all of these parts are intricately connected and need to work together well. Everyone has a urogenital system, but this term is most commonly used to refer to the physically male one.

We talked about how position and restriction can affect the function of the uterus and friends, and the same holds true here. All of those tubes carrying important stuff around need their space! When dysfunction occurs, we can look at a number of potential causes, both physical and emotional. Here are the most common issues to arise:

Benign prostatic hyperplasia (BPH): BPH is a benign (non-cancerous) enlargement of the prostate gland. Conventional thought is that after an initial growth spurt at puberty, the prostate 'normally' starts growing again at around age 25 and continues throughout life, causing 50% of men to develop BPH between ages 51 and 60. But why would the body do that to itself? Another perspective is that excessive sitting (muscle tension/reduced circulation), stress (muscle tension/reduced circulation/stress hormones) and/or overexercise (muscle tension/reduced circulation) causes an overly acidic environment in the pelvis. The body, in its wisdom

to self-regulate, calls for water to dilute the acidity of the prostate, increasing its size. It's just a theory, but I encourage you to keep things moving for this and so many reasons! When the prostate gets bigger than is ideal, it constricts the urethra, which can cause numerous urinary, bladder and even kidney issues.

Prostatitis: This condition comes in different types and can be caused by injury or scar tissue, muscle tension, stress, or prostate stones amongst other potential causes:

◎ **Bacterial prostatitis (acute or chronic):** This is a bacterial infection that requires testing and treatment. If the case is acute, you can have typical infection symptoms, such as fever and chills, and both can cause pain and urinary and sexual function issues. It can be caused by contaminated urine flowing back through the urethra, so you can see how these conditions could be caused by one nother. Bacterial prostatitis is not contagious, but condoms can prevent some infections that can lead to it.

◎ **Chronic prostatitis / Asymptomatic inflammatory prostatitis:** This is an inflammation of the prostate that is not an infection. It can cause pelvic pain, pain with urinary and sexual function, or no symptoms at all. So what is the difference between BPH and non-bacterial prostatitis? Generally, 'enlargement' (as with BPH) happens slowly over time, whereas 'inflammation' ('-itis') occurs more quickly (as with prostatitis). One thing your doctor will keep an eye on in either case is your PSA (prostate-specific antigen) levels, to ensure that there is no underlying cancer.

Prostate stones: These are calcifications that can cause no harm, but can also cause pain and/or prostatitis and make it difficult to clear out an infection or heal inflammation.

Prostate cancer: This type of cancer is much more prevalent after age 40 and is much more treatable if detected early! The symptoms can be all of the ones we already mentioned, along with a dull pain in the low back, pelvis and/or thighs, loss of appetite/weight loss or bone pain. Prostate cancer can metastasize, or spread to other parts of the body.

Testicular cancer: This type of cancer most commonly occurs between the ages of 15 and 44! It is less common than prostate cancer, and very treatable. The symptoms are a palpable (but painless) lump, swelling of a testicle, dull pain in a testis, scrotum or groin, or tenderness in chest/breast tissue and/or low back pain.

Erectile dysfunction: Research, testing and treatment of sexual function issues has been almost completely focused on those who have difficulty with penile erections. But "arousal nonconcordance" can and does happen to every type of person, and the reasons are sometimes physical, but oftentimes emotional and psychological. The clitoris is made up of erectile tissue as well, so the same processes are at play. People with cardiovascular disease, hypertension, diabetes mellitus, tobacco use, hyperlipidemia, hypogonadism, lower urinary tract symptoms, metabolic syndrome, and depression are more likely to have ED...so you can see how it spans across multiple factors! In *Come As You Are*, Emily Nagoski explores in depth the psychological side of what triggers our 'accelerator' or our 'brakes', and how to understand and communicate about it! It does center **cisgender** women, but really has so much wisdom for every person about ourselves and each other.

Fertility issues: Historically, fertility issues have been assumed to be related to womb health and function, but there are many conditions, including all the ones listed above that can lead to the sperm not being set up for success. Additionally, there can be issues with numbers or strength of sperm, thickness of semen, genetic variances in sperm and numerous other possible factors. Fertility challenges can happen to anyone!

THE UROGENITAL SYSTEM

1. KIDNEY (2)
2. ADRENAL GLAND (2)
3. SACRUM
4. BOWEL
5. URETER (2)
6. BLADDER
7. PUBIC BONE
8. PROSTATE GLAND
9. SEMINAL VESICLE (2)
10. BULBOURETHRAL GLAND (2)

11. TESTIS (2)
12. EPIDIDYMIS (2)
13. PENIS
14. SCROTUM

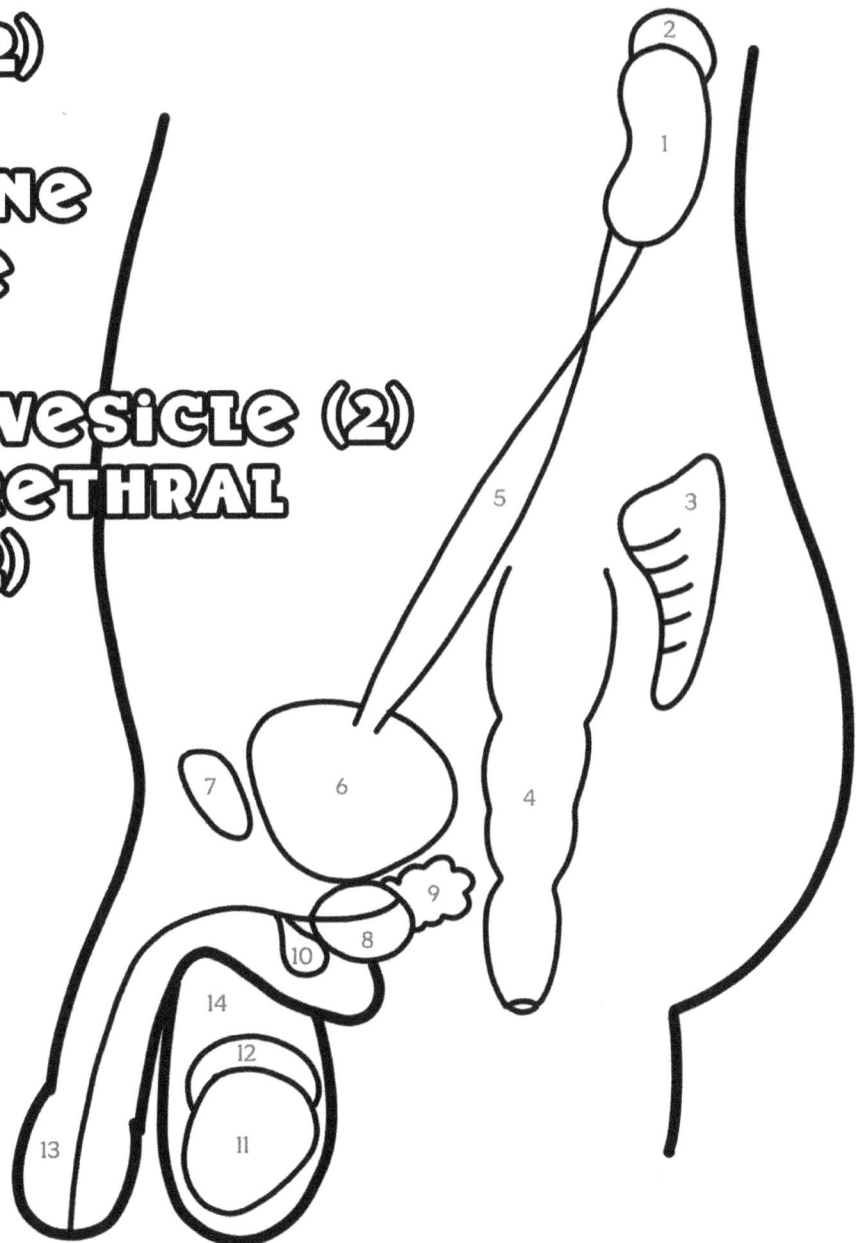

Androgens!

Now we're going to spend some time playing out how these hormones work their magic in your body's systems.

It's a great example of how everything is connected, and how when one piece falls out of line, the whole kit and caboodle can get off track!

Androgens are **steroid hormones,** and the main one at play here is testosterone, although production of this hormone would be nil if it weren't for its **precursors**!

Here is how the amazing prostate-centered system works, all choreographed like a show choir performance. The main thing about this dance, however, is that it is non-stop! The first part of the process, anyways, is churning on-and-on, day and night. It can speed up and slow down with changes in brain activity and metabolism, but it's pretty much a 24/7 party! Woohoo!

Your **hypothalamus**, using a hormone called GnRh, tells the **pituitary** gland to send out the hormones LH and FSH. The LH and FSH make their way to the **testes** to stimulate the production of androgens, including testosterone. Some of the LH goes to the **adrenal glands** (on top of the kidneys) to inspire androgen production there, but much less than in the testes.

Cells inside the seminiferous tubules (inside the testes) transform into sperm under the influence of the androgens—namely, testosterone.

From here, the sperm head up into the **epididymis**, where they mature, or grow up. Millions of sperm are stored in the epididymis, ready to be released into the **vas deferens** should an ejaculatory event present itself!

Because this sperm production system is ongoing and abundant (healthy testes make 1000-5000 sperm cells/minute!), unused sperm will break down and be absorbed by the body.

Once the body signals that it is time to ejaculate, the mature sperm are released into the **vas deferens**, where they make their way to the urethra.

Along the way, they pick up some much-needed supplies in the **seminal vesicles.** These handy little parts produce around 70% of the content of semen. Semen is made up of: fructose for energy, prostaglandins to prevent immune response against the sperm along their way, clotting factors to make semen thick enough to make it all the way to the egg, and an alkaline solution conducive to sperm for the urethra and vagina (those areas are generally more acidic than alkaline).

The prostate is a muscular organ that contracts during ejaculation to both close the opening to the bladder, and to force semen to exit...at ~26mph! It also produces prostatic fluid, which adds bulk to the fluid produced in the seminal vesicles and helps make the perfect thickness to support sperm motility, or the ability to move easily!

The bulbourethral glands produce the first fluid to pass through the urethra during an ejaculatory event. The fluid is mucous-like, which preps the pathway for easy passage of semen, and it also cleans out the urethra of any remaining urine or other cells. The fluid is also called the 'pre-ejaculate', or 'precum'.

Of course, we have been focusing mainly on the *reproductive* process of this event... but there is certainly a recreational one! Not everyone is having sex to make more humans...sometimes it's just for connection and fun! But we still want our bodies working well so it can be a positive experience for everyone. That's the goal, so don't leave your body (or anyone else's, for that matter) behind!

Your body is likely working just fine, but something simple can leave it off kilter. If you are having any symptoms or dysfunction, reach out for help! Document your symptoms so you can provide detailed info to practitioners, do some research (but be aware that self-diagnosis can sometimes go sideways), and get back in the swing of things! Remember that stress can have a huge impact on the function of these processes.

Your urogenital system is super intricate and important, and you don't have to suffer!

Sometimes we just need a little help from our friends and professionals!

ANDROGENS AND FRIENDS

HYPOTHALAMUS

$\Downarrow$

G_NRH

$\Downarrow$

PITUITARY

LH FSH

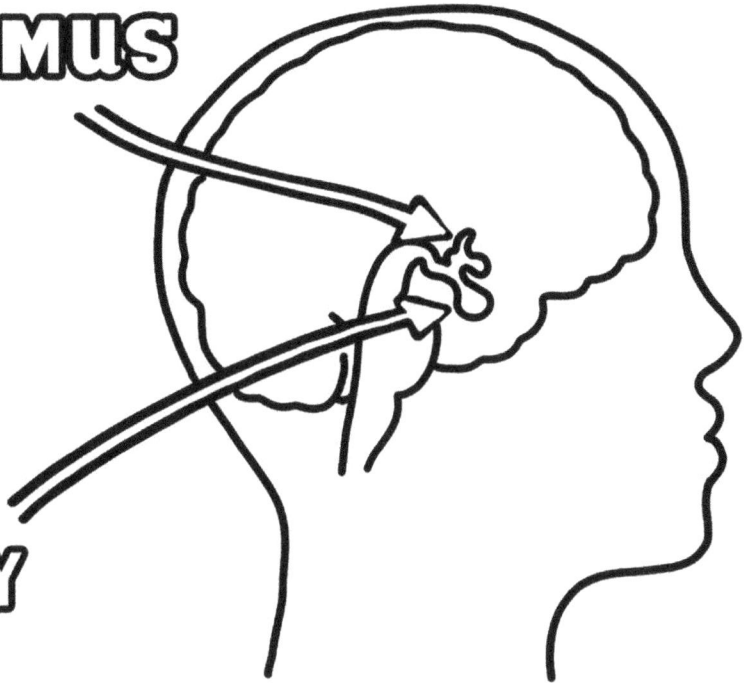

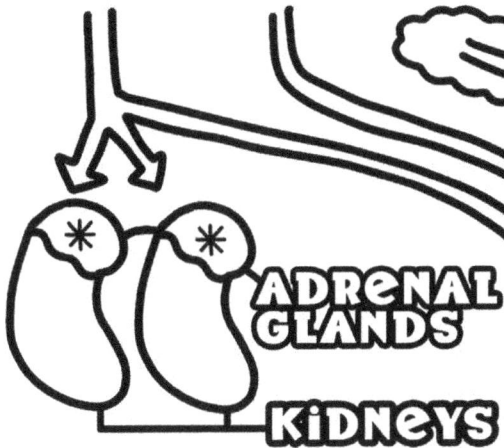

ADRENAL GLANDS

KIDNEYS

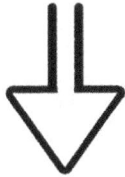 = ANDROGENS

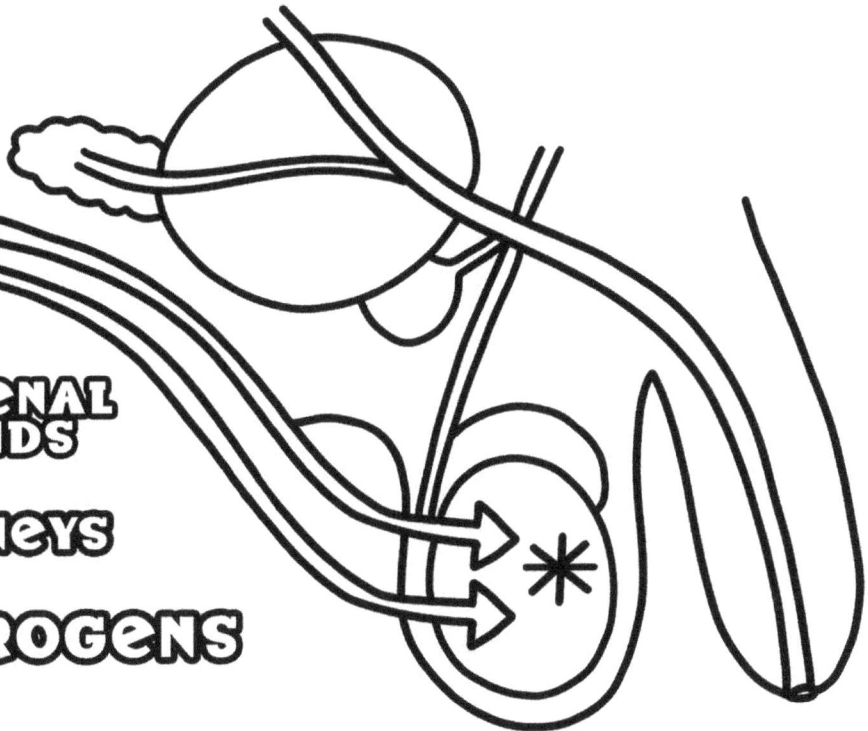

It's a Circle of a Cycle

These graphs show us the basic course of events in a menstrual cycle, and hormones orchestrate all of it! Anywhere from 25 to 35 day cycles are normal, as long as they are a relatively consistent length from month-to-month.[30] Remember that all types of people can menstruate (cisgender girls/women, transgender boys/men, and nonbinary folks)...and all types of people don't!

Here's how a textbook menstrual cycle unfolds throughout one 28-day period:

Days 1-5: Menstruation. The release of endometrial tissue and blood that has built up over the course of the month. During this time, all of your reproductive hormone levels are relatively low. Your uterus will double in weight and size as you approach menses. Remember all of those ligaments keeping it in a good spot? They are particularly sensitive to strain during this time, since the weight of your uterus is about a half a pound! This is a good time to do restful and creative projects...chillax!

Days 6-9: The pituitary gland in our brains starts releasing a hormone called **FSH** (follicle-stimulating hormone), inspiring 15-20 eggs in each ovary to develop, each attempting to reach maturity! Every egg is encased in a follicle which is releasing estrogen in order for ovulation to eventually occur. This can be an energetic time, and a good one to get back into your exercise and other active self-care routines!

Days 10-11: Continuing the follicular phase (the egg-maturing part), both FSH and estrogen are in full swing. The increase in estrogen is causing the endometrial lining of the uterus to thicken, preparing it to receive a fertilized egg and making your **cervical mucus** more slippery (conducive to sperm travel and sex). At the end of this time, we experience a burst of LH (luteinizing hormone) which, along with the FSH, stimulates and completes egg growth.

Days 12-17: Ovulation. Once your body reaches an estrogen threshold, a burst of LH is triggered and the most mature egg wins (two eggs released could result in fraternal twins and one egg that splits in two would result in identical twins). The egg is released, and it can take as little as 20 seconds for the fimbria of your fallopian tubes to draw it in for the journey to your uterus. Your endometrium is cozy and ready to host, your cervix/uterus is set high inside, inviting spermy visitors with optimally slippery cervical fluid. You are fertile. The egg will last about 6-24 hours once it's released. If the egg is not fertilized, it disintegrates and is either absorbed by the body or exits with your menstrual flow. The released egg can be fertilized by sperm that just arrived, or that have been hanging around for as many as 5 days! So... if you ovulate on day 14, fertilization can occur with a sperm that has been there since day 9. Predicting this window is possible when you have a regular cycle, but more difficult when you don't.

Days 18-22: The follicle (sac) that your egg ruptured from has transformed itself into a **corpus luteum**, which is releasing progesterone, a heat producing hormone, to nourish and sustain the endometrium (if fertilization and pregnancy occur, it will continue to do so until the placenta takes over to nourish the growing fetus until childbirth). Progesterone will cause your body temperature to rise, so you might notice being more heat-intolerant during this time. Your endometrial lining is building up with nutrients and ideal conditions to prepare for an incoming egg. Time to cool off in that lake, river or pool!

Days 23-26: Your endometrium has reached its pinnacle of fullness (5-6mm); nutrients are flowing in through a proliferation of vessels and life-sustaining capacities are at their most abundant...you are full of the good stuff! Your body is working hard to make all of this happen, so it is a good time to nourish yourself, get quality rest...put the 'to-do' list aside for some connecting activities, whether on your own or with friends and family.

Day 27: And...progesterone drops the mic. That is, assuming no pregnancy has occurred. After a dramatic swell of supply, your corpus luteum stops producing this pregnancy-supporting hormone. The lack of progesterone and **HCG (human chorionic gonadotropin**, released by a fertilized ovum in the uterus) cause the endometrial wall to start breaking down, and in the next 24 hours or so, your menses begin. Healthy menstruation is bright red from beginning to end, with little to no discomfort (not what pain relief companies have tried to teach us)! Teenage cycles can be a bit more troublesome and irregular, but diet, exercise and stress play a *huge* role!

Another way to look at this is to separate out the two main areas of physical change throughout the month: the uterine cycle and the ovarian cycle. The second coloring sheet will show you this perspective:

1. **Luteinizing Hormone**
2. **Estrogen**
3. **Progesterone**
4. **Follicle Stimulating Hormone**

Pretty flippin' magical, right?!

CIRCLE ⊙ CYCLE

cd1

MENSES

cd5

FOLLICULAR

cd9

LUTEAL

cd21

EGG TRAVEL TIME

cd14

F*

OVULATION

FERTILE WINDOW

FERTILE

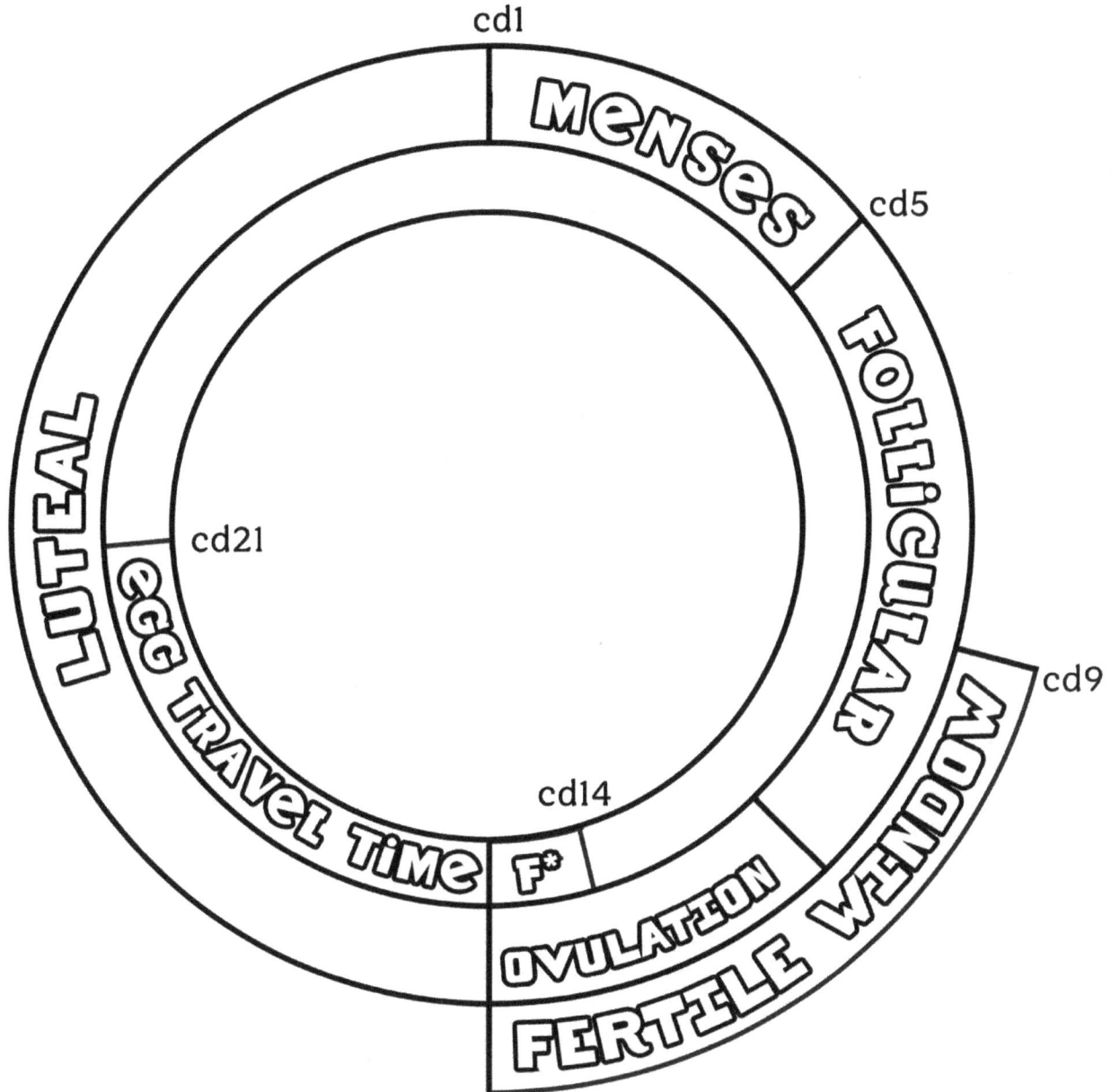

CD = CYCLE DAY
F* = FERTILIZATION
(FERTILE WINDOW: APPROXIMATE!)

TWO HORMONE FLOWS

UTERINE CYCLE:

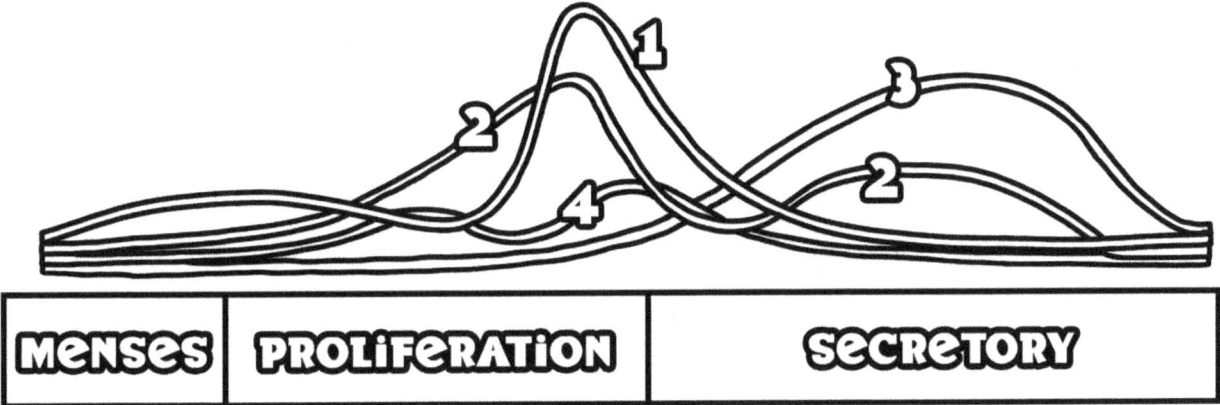

MENSES	PROLIFERATION	SECRETORY

OVARIAN CYCLE:

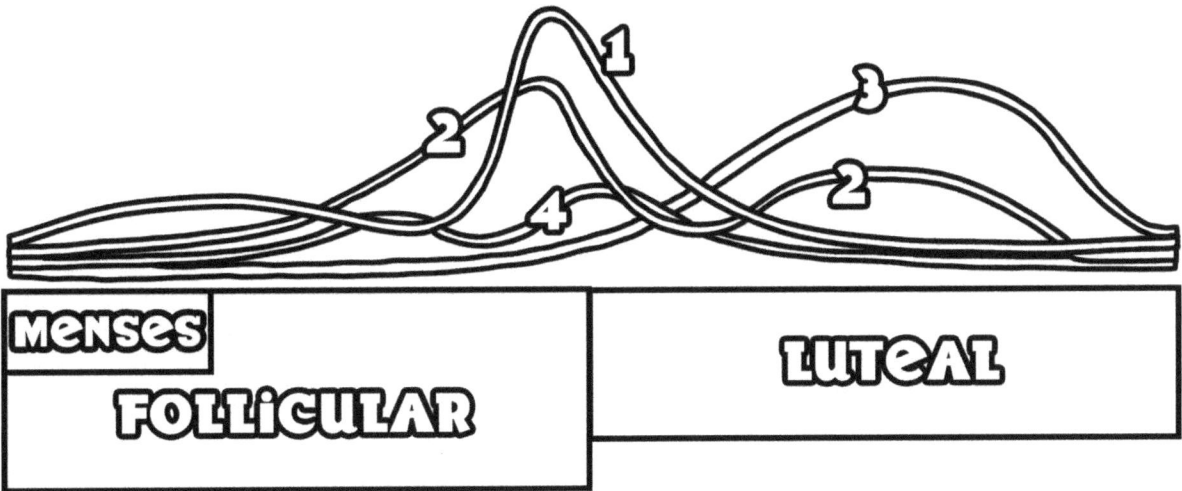

MENSES		LUTEAL
FOLLICULAR		

We Are All One

Now we are going to go wayyyyyy back... back to when you were mere cells waiting for instructions. It is amazing how it all happened...just like you!

In the beginning, our cells were all the same:

The genital tubercle are the cells that eventually form either the clitoris or the penis.

The labioscrotal swellings are the cells that eventually become either the labia or the scrotum.

The gonads are the cells that eventually become either the ovaries or the testes.

Eventually, we will see that the elements causing these individual developments are numerous and vary greatly...but for now let's let our *sameness* amaze us![31]

Let's learn a bit more about each structure:

- **Clitoris** (top left): This sometimes-elusive bundle of 8,000 nerve endings is mostly internal, but is no less sensitive than its external counterpart, the penis. Straddling the vaginal canal, it is actually made up of erectile tissue...which means it has erections, too!

- **Labia majora, minora, and mons pubis** (top right): These three sections form the outer portion of the vulva. Commonly mistaken for the vagina (which is internal),

they make a cozy home for the very important parts and processes within!

- **Penis, scrotum, and testes** (bottom left): We just went over these in detail, but let's add that the abundant nerves cover not only the penis, but also the scrotum...which you probably know if you have one!

- **Uterus and ovaries** (bottom right): Also something we know lots about, but isn't it amazing that all of these parts were made of the same materials?!

EMBRYONIC SEX DIFFERENTIATION

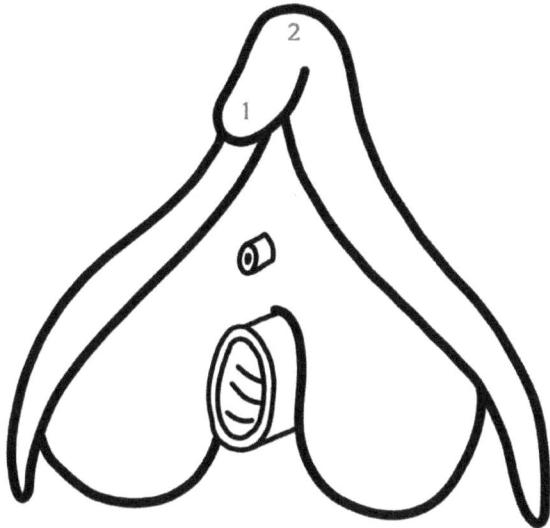

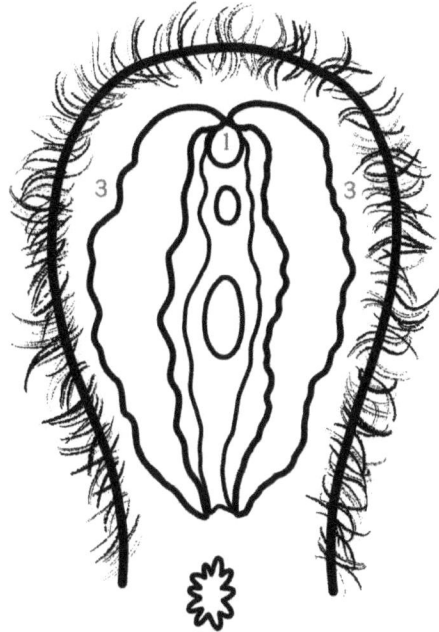

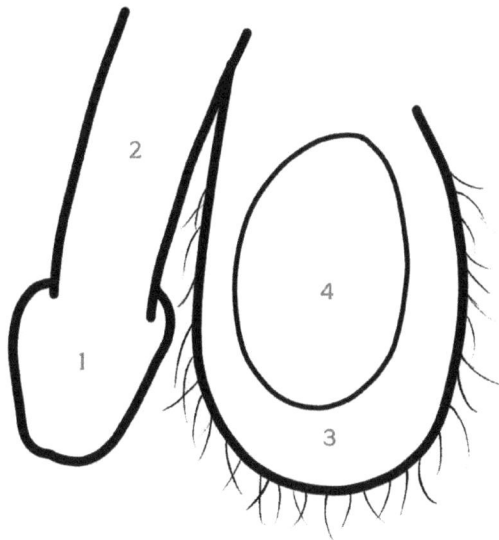

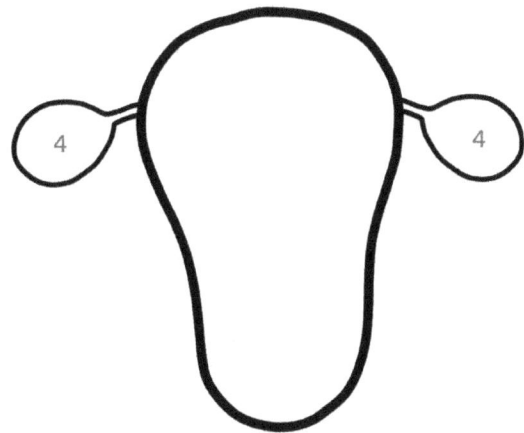

1. GLANS OF CLITORIS/PENIS
2. SHAFT OF CLITORIS/PENIS
3. LABIA MAJORA/SCROTUM
4. OVARIES/TESTES

We Are All Unique

Okay, now we're going to get *real* technical.

Stick with me, because the results will be well worth the effort! While there are lots of ways that we are similar or the same, there is also an array of (possibly surprising) things that make us very diverse...and that's a good thing!

So what happens to us, scientifically, to determine our sex?

First of all, let's differentiate between sex and gender:

Sex is science. It is all of the many physiological processes that make our cells do what they do, which varies greatly! When we look at the science of sex, it will become clear that the binary (only two options) does not represent reality.

Gender is identity. We are not talking about gender when we are talking about sex. Gender identity is one's personal feeling and expression of themselves. It can change over time, and can look like a rainbow of things. We are not focused on gender in this scientific exploration.

Here are the elements at play as your cells are differentiating, or expressing themselves. *Note: this is a simplification of a very complex process:*

1. Chromosomes are what we hear about most when people talk about (biological) sex: the Xs and the Ys. For many years now, we have simply thought: XX = female and XY = male. But we can't really talk about chromosomes without also talking about *genes* (not jeans). Chromosomes carry our genetic information, or our genes.

The most valuable gene when it comes to biological sex is the SRY gene.

The SRY gene *most commonly* hangs out on the Y chromosome, and is part of what triggers a fetus to develop a penis, scrotum and testes. But sometimes there is no SRY gene on an XY pair, causing someone to be *chromosomally male but genetically and physically female*. This person would traditionally be **assigned female at birth**, but it's more complicated than that.

Another option is for the SRY gene to be contained in an X chromosome (on either an XX or an XY pair of chromosomes). If the person has an XY paired chromosome, they would be *chromosomally and genetically male*, but *physically female*. If it was an XX pair, they would be *chromosomally* and *physically female, but genetically male.* You can also be born with two Xs and a Y (XXY), which would result in being **assigned male at birth**, but with variations in hormone levels and the size, shape and appearance of genitals and secondary sex characteristics.[32]

2. Genes code for hormones and hormones regulate genes. They are thick as thieves, but they do not follow a binary formula! This means that hormone levels can vary greatly, both during fetal development, and later during puberty and beyond. Given the wide array of chromosomal and genetic possibilities, assuming the range of what a 'normal' hormone level is for an individual is inaccurate. As we learn more, that word 'normal' becomes less relevant.[33]

3. Hormone cell receptors are substances in and on cells that bind to hormones. The hormones tell the cell how to act. They 'turn on' the processes of the cell at certain times, and for certain periods of time. But sometimes those receptors don't work! This can affect development, appearance and the function of some systems and structures.[34]

So basically, you could be chromosomally, genetically, physically and/or hormonally female, male or intersex. Some of these manifestations of us are apparent at birth, some don't show up until puberty or adulthood...and many people will never know they had some of the many possible options of humanhood! It is really quite cool and liberating, right?

Much of this research and experience has been coming out of the **intersex** community. The definition of intersex is very broad, and different based on who you ask. *"Nature doesn't decide where the category of "male" ends and the category of "intersex" begins, or where the category of "intersex" ends and the category of "female" begins. Humans decide." ~The Intersex Society of North America*[35]

A lot of trauma and damage has been done to make babies fit into the binary by surgically altering them before they have had a chance to define themselves. Intersex and transgender rights advocates have been hard at work and speaking up, putting their lives on the line... teaching us a lesson we should take into all areas of life:

What makes us different makes us stronger and better!

1. CHROMOSOMES AND their GENES

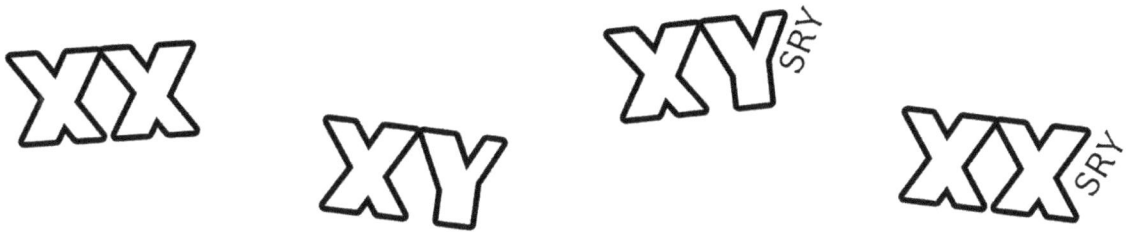

XX

XY

XY SRY

XX SRY

2. GENES AND their HORMONES

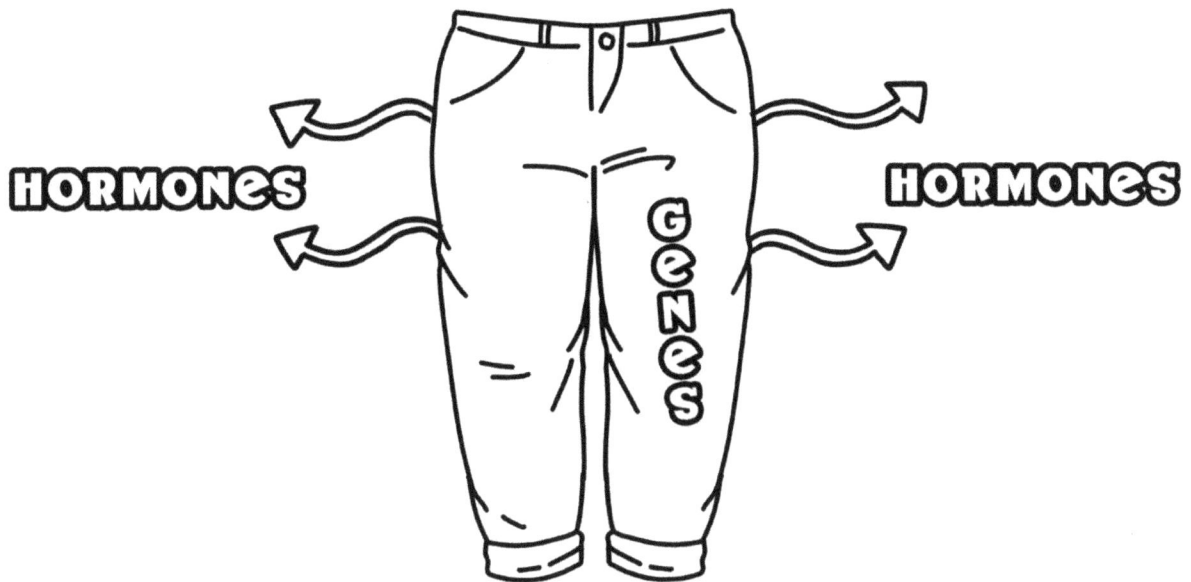

HORMONES

GENES

HORMONES

3. HORMONE CELL RECEPTORS

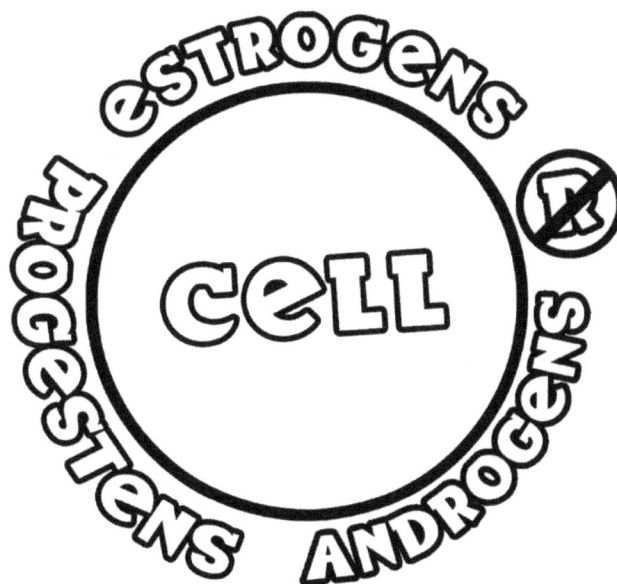

ESTROGENS

PROGESTENS

CELL

ANDROGENS

Hormonal Interventions and Other Preventions!

Now you know how the body is trying to operate in a variety of scenarios. Let's talk about options for steering the ship, so to speak. Sometimes you don't want your body to do things it's doing (or you want it to do things it isn't!).

The important thing is that you research what the method you're considering is trying to accomplish in your body, and be aware of any potential side effects or contraindications. Knowledge is power! Sometimes the physiological or psychological benefits outweigh the potential risks, but it's important to have all of the information before you make a decision for your body.

- **Hormonal birth control:** The birth control pill, patch, ring, implant, shot, and hormonal IUD (intrauterine device). All are designed to disallow pregnancy, but are also used to ease painful menstrual cramps, address heavy bleeding, facilitate a fertility treatment or support a transgender/non-binary person. Most do this by preventing ovulation. The birth control pill was *re*-designed as a marketing strategy to mimic a normal cycle, allowing you to "menstruate" once/month (called 'withdrawal bleeding'), but that bleeding is not an actual menstruation, as no uterine lining was triggered to build up. Some versions don't fluctuate the hormone dose (no sugar pills), and so don't cause withdrawal bleeding. They do have low-dose options that don't include the synthetic estrogen and are designed to allow ovulation but still prevent pregnancy (50-60% of people still don't ovulate on this pill or the IUD version). Birth/menstrual control is a personal choice, and unwanted pregnancies are life-changing, so weigh the options with people you trust! Big pharma doesn't always have your best interest in mind, so *you* have to...which isn't to say you shouldn't use them, but with eyes wide open! Ovulation is healthy, so don't give it up if you don't have to!

- **IUD (intrauterine device):** This is a device inserted into the uterus designed to prevent pregnancy. The hormonal type acts as a hormonal birth control would. There is also a copper (hormone-free) version that acts by keeping the lining of your uterus irritated, making it inhospitable to a fertilized egg.

- **Fertility enhancing drugs:** The opposite of birth control! There are many options that guide a cycle to achieve a healthy pregnancy when the body is struggling to do so, or the parent(s) are single, same-sexed, or unable to for some other reason.

- **Hormone therapy:** Transgender people sometimes choose to take hormones, under the care of a doctor. People also use hormone therapy during a difficult transition into menopause, after an oophorectomy (removal of the ovaries) and increasing numbers of people are being diagnosed with low testosterone, which causes difficult symptoms that can be alleviated through HRT (hormone replacement therapy).

- **Vasectomy/tubal ligation:** Birth control surgeries. In a vasectomy, the vas deferens is cut to disallow sperm from mixing with the other components of semen, so that fertilization won't occur. This is an outpatient surgery and it is usually reversible. A tubal ligation cuts and ties the fallopian tubes so the egg can't reach the uterus.

- **No sex:** Well, there are tons of ways to have sex, and not all of them risk pregnancy and/or STIs! Knowing when, what and how to touch (and not) is a good way to be an empowered sexual being...if and when you want to!

- **Levonorgestrel:** "the morning after pill". Emergency contraception that either (or both) prevents ovulation or fertilization. It needs to be taken by 72 hours after unprotected (or failed barrier-method) sex and should not be taken on a regular basis for health reasons.

- **PrEP (pre-exposure prophylaxis):** A pill taken daily to prevent exposure to HIV. There is another version (**PEP**) that can be taken in the event you have been exposed. *PrEP/Pep do NOT prevent any OTHER sexually transmitted infections!*

- **Fertility awareness method:** A shout out goes to this old school/new school way to either prevent or achieve pregnancy, but also to identify health issues. Your menstrual cycle tells you A LOT about your overall health! The three factors you track are: basal (waking) body temperature, cervical mucus and cervical position. Practice this method before you rely on it for birth control and know that an irregular cycle is much harder to rely on (but can give you good information for your practitioner if you are having concerns). Hormonal birth control makes this method inaccurate, since the body is not cycling like it normally would.

These complex choices are very important and personal. Remember that marketing is a powerful force in shaping our perceptions, as well as societal, community, friend and family pressures...**You do you!**

BODY AUTONOMY AND YOUR HEALTH

FERTILITY AWARENESS

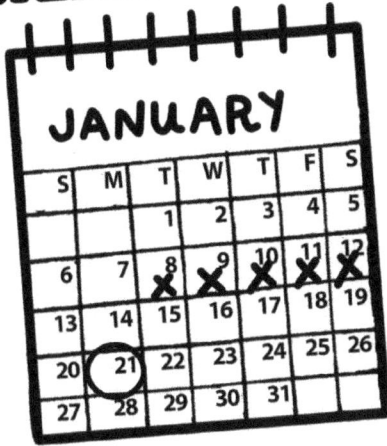

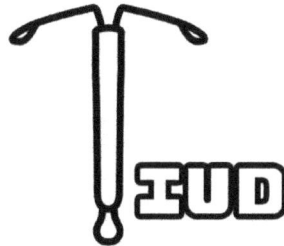

IUD

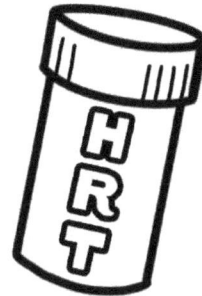

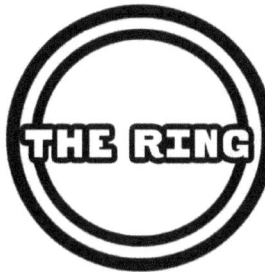

THE RING

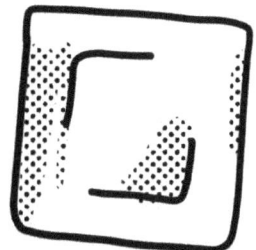

THE PATCH

NO ✕ SEX

VASECTOMY

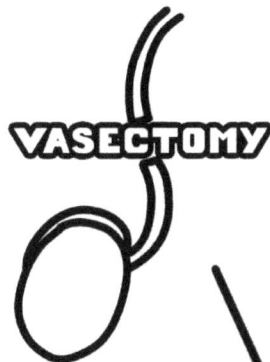

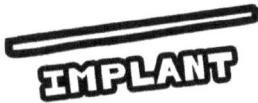

IMPLANT

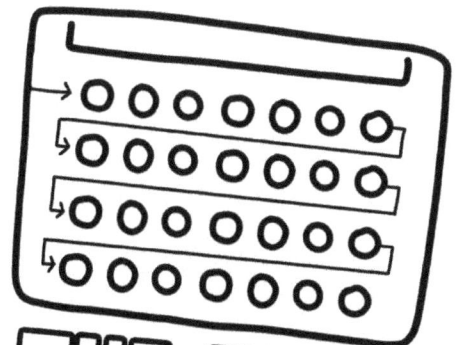

THE PILL

LEVONORGESTREL

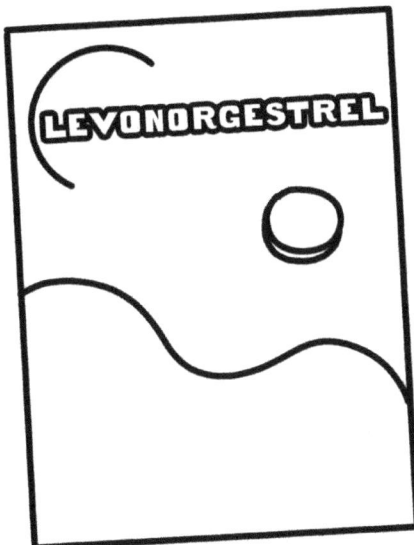

SHOT

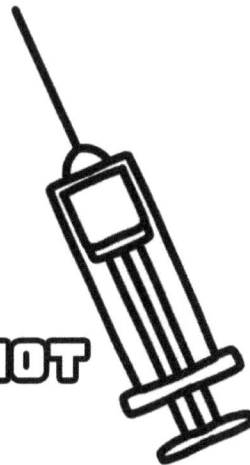

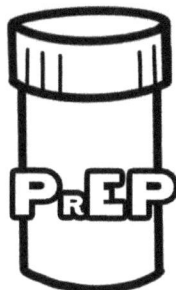

PrEP

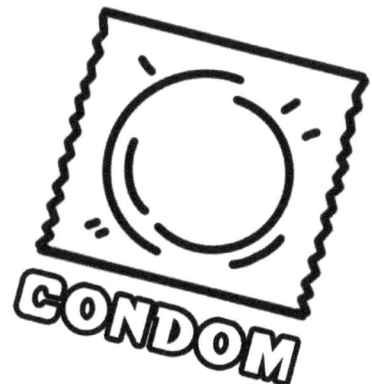

CONDOM

STIs (aka STDs):

Condoms deserve their very own coloring page. All hail the mighty condom!

We will be learning about some of the different varieties of sexually transmitted infections. Let me point out that condoms are *the only* option designed to prevent both pregnancy *and* infection (when used correctly)!

There are other barrier methods, such as the diaphragm, cervical cap, 'female' condom and spermicidal foam, sponges, and dental dams, but the condom, made in multiple sizes for all of the different penises around, comes in at 98% effective at preventing most STIs and pregnancies. Some STIs are transmitted skin-to-skin, so are not covered by condoms (literally).

A dental dam is a barrier method for use with oral sex to help prevent STI transmission. It's important to think about all the ways that STIs can be passed between us, including all the different ways that we have sex! Testing and treatment are an irreplaceable part of sexual health, both for you and those you have sex with.

Chlamydia is a common bacterial infection transmitted through vaginal, anal or oral sex. Untreated, it can cause a serious infection in the womb which can be life threatening and cause fertility issues. It can also be transmitted to a baby during childbirth. Antibiotics are the remedy. **Prevention**: using condoms or dental dams. **Symptoms**: burning sensation while urinating, abnormal discharge from vagina, penis or anus, pain or swelling in one or both testicles, rectal pain or bleeding. Sometimes there are no symptoms.

Gonorrhea is a common bacterial infection. It is spread through vaginal, anal or oral sex. Untreated, it can cause a serious infection in the womb which can be life threatening and cause fertility issues. It can also be transmitted to a baby during childbirth. Antibiotics are the remedy. **Prevention**: using condoms or dental dams. **Symptoms**: Painful or burning sensation while urinating, white, yellow or green discharge from penis, abnormal discharge from vagina or anus, swollen or painful testicles, vaginal bleeding in between periods, anal itching, soreness, bleeding or painful bowel movements. Often there are no symptoms.

Human papillomavirus (HPV) is the most common STI. 4 out of 5, or 80% of sexually active people get HPV at some point in their lives.[36] It is spread through skin-to-skin contact and can affect the genitals, mouth and throat. Usually, HPV goes away on its own, but sometimes it can lead to cancer or genital warts. The strains of HPV that cause warts are not the same strains that can lead to cancer. Genital warts can be removed by a doctor, and there are many treatments for the cancer-causing strains. Regular testing and treatment is the remedy. **Prevention**: using condoms or dental dams. **Most people have no symptoms.**

Herpes is a very common virus that affects the mouth and/or genitals. More than half of Americans have oral herpes, and 1 in 6 have genital herpes. Herpes is transmitted through skin-to-skin contact of the mouth and/or genitals. There is no cure, but learning what triggers outbreaks for you can help reduce and minimize frequency and duration. They can flare up during times of stress or illness and there are medications that can help. **Prevention**: avoiding contact at the first symptoms of a sore and using condoms and dental dams. **Symptoms**: painful, blistering sores that can start with numbness, tingling, itching, discoloration.

Syphilis is a common bacterial infection that is transmitted through sex. It can affect the genitals, anus and sometimes the lips and mouth. **Prevention**: the use of condoms and dental dams. Testing and treatment are imperative! **Symptoms**: (usually painless) sores on the vagina, anus, penis or scrotum that can be treated very effectively with antibiotics. Untreated, it can cause serious damage, such as brain damage, paralysis and blindness!

Trichomoniasis (trich) is a parasite transmitted through sexual fluids of the penis and vagina. It is the most common curable STI. Most often, it does not cause symptoms, so people don't know they have it. **Prevention**: condoms! When present, the **symptoms** are vaginitis, which is an irritation of the vulva and/or vagina. It can also infect your urethra, resulting in irritation, smelly discharge, and painful or frequent peeing. Trich is easily treated with medicine.

HIV and AIDS: HIV is the virus that *can* cause AIDS. Not everyone with HIV has AIDS. HIV can damage your immune system, and left untreated, can result in AIDS. In the US, there are around 1.1 million people living with HIV, and around 38,000 new infections happen per year. While HIV/AIDS is not curable, there are very effective medications so the person can avoid ever progressing to AIDS. HIV is transmitted through vaginal and anal sex, by sharing needles or accidentally getting stuck with a needle, or by getting blood or sexual fluids into an open cut on your body. The symptoms can take many years to develop, so prevention, testing and treatment are imperative. **Prevention**: we talked about PrEP/PEP as a medical preventative, but condoms and dental dams are also preventative.

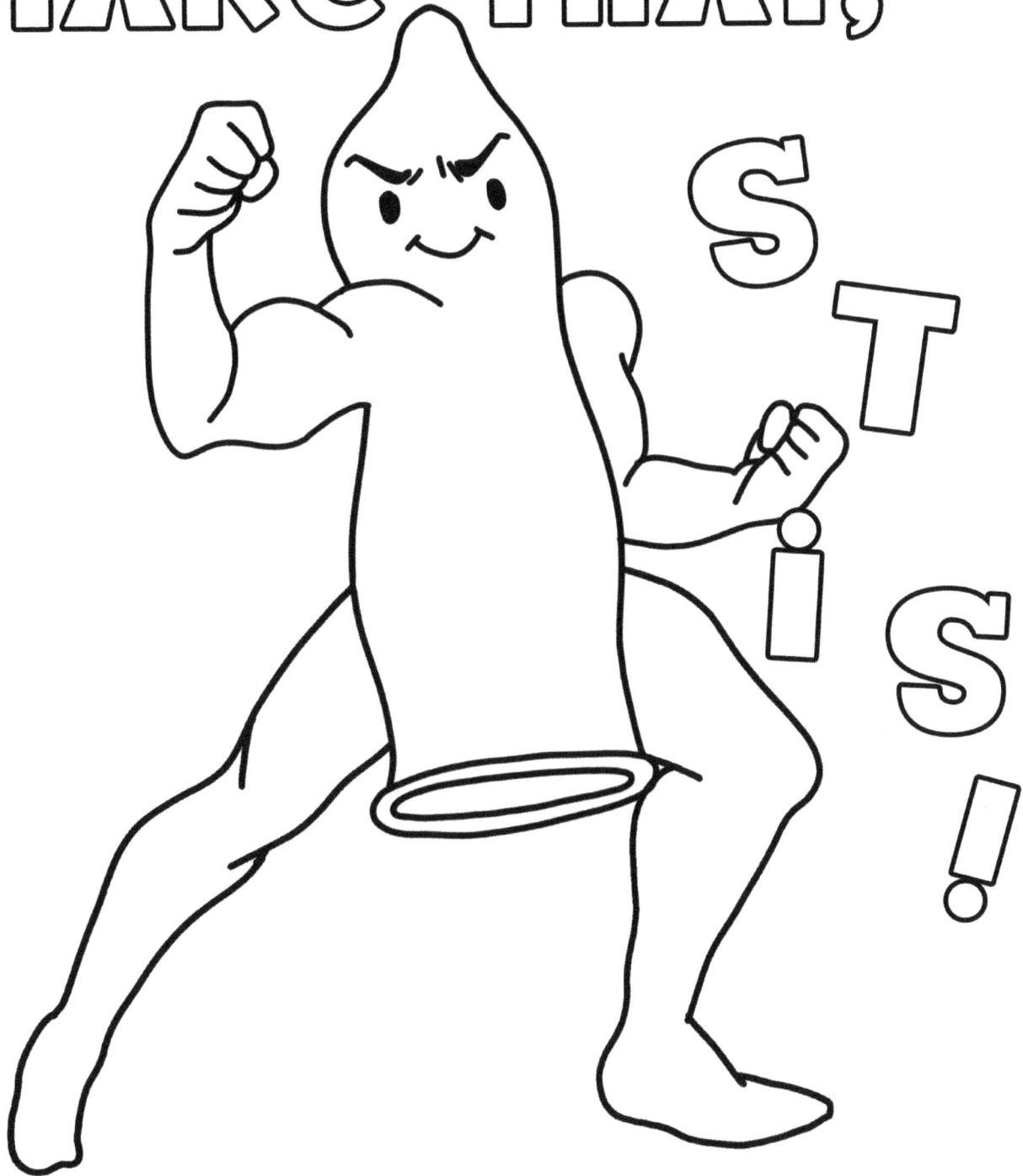

A is for Awkward, O is for Oxytocin

We're going to switch gears here and talk about a common human emotion, and one of the hormones that drives, and overrides it! We are social creatures who want to connect...but why can it feel *so awkward?!* Another term for awkwardness is social anxiety. *Some* levels of social anxiety cause too much suffering and need professional support, but some amount of nervousness is normal. I find it important, when judging ourselves, to remember how we would see or advise a friend if they were going through the very same thing...be a good friend to yourself! On some level, we're all just bumbling around trying to be loved and accepted.

There is a *lot* we don't know about how emotions play out in the body, but here are some of the things happening when we connect with others', most often all at once!

- The parts of the brain most involved in our body's emotional reactions are the frontal lobe and the amygdala. The frontal lobe mostly reacts to happiness and pleasure, while the amygdala is focused on anger, fear and sadness. But which is awkwardness? It can be both! Doesn't flirting sometimes feel like both fear *and* pleasure?

- Normal (or not-so-normal) fluctuations in sex hormones can make you feel more or less anxious. Puberty, the changes during a menstrual cycle, menopause and of course our general emotional state can intensify our interpersonal experiences.

- When we notice (or remember) ourselves acting awkwardly, it activates the pain center in the brain, producing that 'cringe' feeling.

We can see how the intensity we are feeling is caused by (and is causing) changes in our bodies. But what can we do to help ourselves feel better? Beyond acknowledging our common human experience, all of the general things you do to keep yourself healthy can help (diet, sleep, exercise), having close connections to family, friends and pets and trying stress-reduction techniques like yoga and meditation.

Talk to people about how you are feeling, giggle with them about each other's less-than-graceful moments and get help if it feels overwhelming or debilitating. We are here to connect with each other! So let's make sure we can.

*CUE UP THE CHEESY TUNES . . . now we're going to talk about love.

I am not here to define love in its entirety... let's leave it somewhat undefinable, to retain the *magic.* *Why* you are attracted to *who* you are attracted to falls mostly in the realm of psychology...it has a lot to do with your life experiences and role models. But there is also specific brain science happening! Let's take a look at a general breakdown:

Lust: Activated by our imagination, testosterone and estrogen join forces to make us *want* to engage intimately with others, sometimes even before there is an object of our affection...unless that object is ourselves! It all begins in the brain.

Attraction/infatuation: Dopamine (a neurotransmitter) and norepinephrine (its hormonal counterpart) start firing and flowing, causing us to feel giddy, nervous, excited and energized all at once. They act on the reward centers in the brain, so the dance of flirtation is led by these chemicals. The reward we seek is attention, and the brain will inspire us to be brave to get it! This phase is also associated with a decrease in serotonin levels, which, interestingly, is also found in people with obsessive-compulsive disorder. This can be why we are so focused on the object of our desire! These are powerful chemicals, and are very similar to what happens to the brain on cocaine...highly addictive! It can overpower our conscious mind because it feels so good! If we take this stage slowly, we can avoid even *more* awkwardness later if it doesn't work out. Try to enjoy the little things, even if it's hard not to get swept away on Hormone River! You will do it differently each time as you learn.

Pair-bonding, or 'love': Oxytocin is the hormone that is most commonly thought of as the 'love hormone'. We can see it's more complicated than that, but oxytocin *is* special in that it is not specific only to romantic or sexual bonding. It is released in large amounts during childbirth, and afterwards during breastfeeding. It is released anytime you bond with anyone, be that your friend, your pet, or your sweetheart. Along with the **neuropeptide** vasopressin, it supports long-term bonding. It is very important to have these connections, even if they aren't romantic. It's also similar to the experience of certain drugs, and can be both wonderful and healthy, but sometimes also cause us to override logic and pair-bond with someone who is not right for us!

Heartbreak: During a separation or break-up, corticotropin-releasing hormone is triggered by the hypothalamus, causing the acute distress and longer-term depression of a breakup. When we experience separation from our love, whether temporary or final, it causes us stress, including fear, jealousy, sadness and anger. This can happen whether-or-not the relationship was in our best interest. Self-care is the remedy.

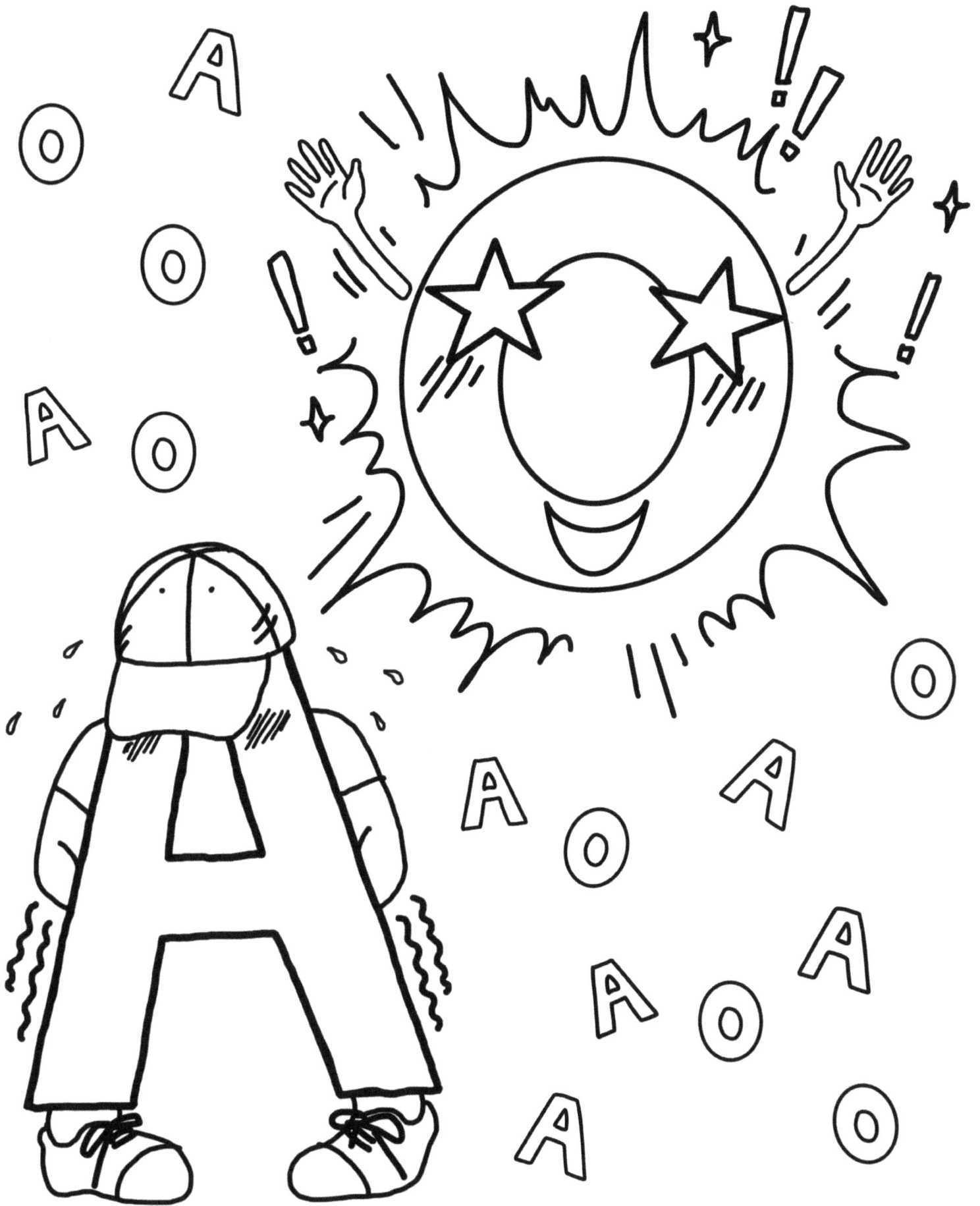

Consent and Rejection

Talking to people about how you feel, what you do and don't want and what you like and don't like can be hard! Saying "no" can be difficult for people of all ages. Our fear of rejection and vulnerability is real. But we can't really have true connection without the ability to be honest with ourselves and others...and it takes practice!

By now you have likely heard the phrase, 'the language of consent'. On the surface, it seems pretty simple: No means no and yes means yes. But there is a *whole lotta* in-between. The reality is: only a CLEAR YES is consent. Everything else is not.

The trickiest part about navigating consent can be *non-verbal* communication. Whether you want to say yes or no, speaking words can be vulnerable, so often we don't. But what does the silence mean, and how might it be interpreted?

We need to take a moment to talk about trauma. People can experience trauma in many forms in their lives—physical, emotional, mental, sexual, institutional, societal, generational. Trauma can manifest in many ways, but one way is the inability to speak or move during moments of fear or anxiety... this is the 'freeze' stress response. Many things can trigger this. If someone you're with gets triggered and freezes, it doesn't mean you've done something wrong, but the ability to stop and change course makes everyone safer and more trusted. It might be vulnerable to stop and ask someone how they are feeling and what they need to feel safe, but it's the right thing to do! If you or someone you care about struggle with the effects of trauma, it can be truly healing and supportive to educate yourself on how trauma works and how to be a good ally.

One of the biggest lessons to learn in life, whether in romantic or platonic situations is this: not hearing or respecting someone's boundaries #isnotlove. Be curious and open...rarely does someone else think or process in the same way as we do!

Rejection is a part of life! But that doesn't make it easy. Practice saying and hearing 'no' with some friends...make a goofy game out of it if that helps, but know that there will be real moments when you will need to either get out of a situation, or avoid being a jerk by asking, listening and respecting.

So, to make things clear:

- **How many responses on this coloring page are consent?** Just one: 'YES!'

- **Is it okay to change my mind?** Yes!

- **Is it okay for someone I am with to change their mind?** Yes!

- **If someone has consented previously, does that mean they are consenting again?** NO! People feel differently in different moments for various reasons...get consent!

- **Is it okay to lie to get out of an uncomfortable or dangerous situation?** Yes!

- **Is it a good idea to let at least one person know where you are and to have them check on you?** Yes! Make a buddy system at parties and on dates.

- **Am I responsible for someone else's experience?** When it comes to consent, yes! You are responsible to make sure that the other person is consenting.

- **Can saying 'no' actually make a relationship better?** Yes! Honesty and vulnerability make a connection stronger. And if it doesn't...byeeeeeee!

- **Is someone in a position to give consent when they have been drinking alcohol?** No. Alcohol and drugs quickly reduce inhibitions, making it likely someone will do something they wouldn't otherwise. You don't want to be the kind of person who takes advantage of that situation, even if you've been drinking/drugging too.

- **Can a minor legally consent to an adult?** No.

- **Can you get consent from someone you are in a position of power over?** No. Students cannot consent to teachers, athletes can't consent to coaches, employees can't consent to bosses, inmates can't consent to corrections officers. The person in the position of power is responsible not to abuse it by engaging romantically or sexually.

- **If someone says 'no' to you, what's your next move?** Respect. They did you a favor by being honest, even if it was hard to hear. Move on, friend.

I know all of this seems obvious, but when emotions are running high, we can get caught in our own fears and desires. Slowing down and asking questions is the best way to learn about someone. Eventually, you will develop enough trust to read their non-verbal communication, but that takes time and practice. It's much better to be the person who asks a lot of questions, than the one who ignores the grey areas out of their own fear or disregard. Connection should feel good to everyone!

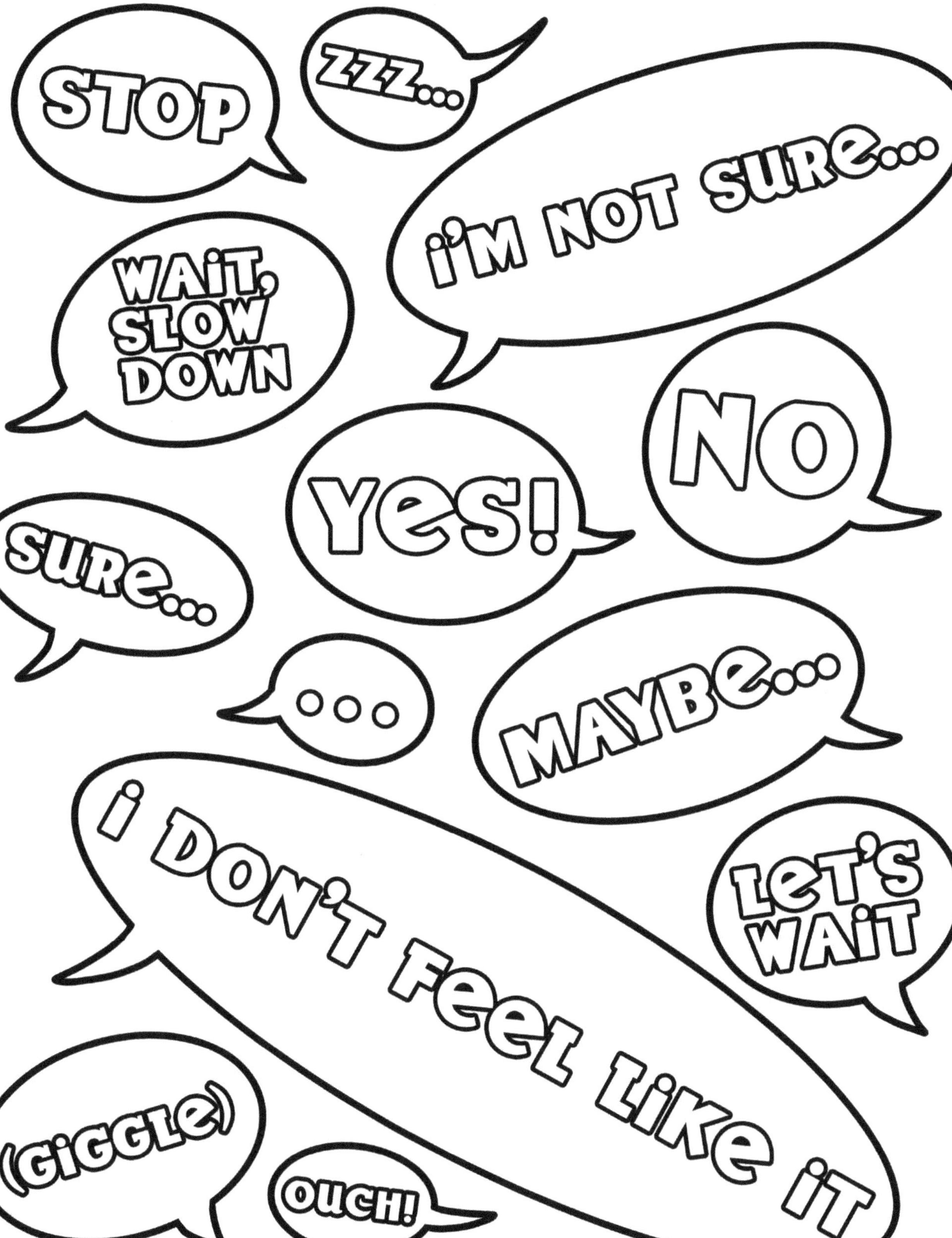
STOP
ZZZ...
I'M NOT SURE...
WAIT, SLOW DOWN
NO
YES!
SURE...
...
MAYBE...
I DON'T FEEL LIKE IT
LET'S WAIT
(GIGGLE)
OUCH!

Stress and Your Health

Let's talk about stress, babes.

Stress is actually a biological imperative, meaning we need the body's natural stress response to survive or escape dangerous or difficult situations. But it should be a temporary state, not a chronic one. Here is a basic rundown of the stress response:

- Once the body decides something is stressful (whether we are aware of it or not), the hypothalamus gets triggered.

- The hypothalamus messages the pituitary gland which then messages the adrenal glands (on top of the kidneys).

- The pituitary releases **adrenocorticotropic hormone** (ACTH), which causes:

- The adrenal glands to release **corticosteroid** (cortisol).

- Cortisol does a number of things, including stimulating the release of **glucose** from the liver (for energy) and acting as an anti-inflammatory (in case of injury).

- A specific part of the adrenal glands called the adrenal medulla is also messaged by the hypothalamus to produce **adrenaline**.

- Adrenaline increases heart rate and blood pressure (the sympathetic nervous system) while simultaneously decreasing functions such as digestion (the parasympathetic nervous system).

So, all of that is groovy... a healthy functioning stress response is a good thing! Also, the 'stressor' can be a positive thing, like the excitement of winning an award, dancing in public, or other moments of nervousness for something good! In this context, stress is an ask of the body to be very active and alert.

Chronic stress, on the other hand, literally causes disease, as well as reduces your quality of life. Let's take a look at this study by NCBI about stress and illness:

"The relationship between stress and illness is complex. The susceptibility to stress varies from person to person. Among the factors that influenced the susceptibility to stress are genetic vulnerability, coping style, type of personality and social support. Not all stress has a negative effect. Studies have shown that short-term stress boosted the immune system, but chronic stress has a significant effect on the immune system that ultimately manifests an illness.

It raises catecholamine and suppressor T cells levels, which suppress the immune system. This suppression in turn raises the risk of viral infection. Stress also leads to the release of histamine, which can trigger severe broncho-constriction in asthmatics. Stress increases the risk for diabetes mellitus, especially in overweight individuals, since psychological stress alters insulin needs. Stress also alters the acid concentration in the stomach, which can lead to peptic ulcers, stress ulcers or ulcerative colitis. Chronic stress can also lead to plaque buildup in the arteries (atherosclerosis), especially if combined with a high-fat diet and sedentary living....There is no scientific evidence of a direct cause-and-effect relationship between the immune system changes and the development of cancer. However, recent studies found a link between stress, tumour development and suppression of natural killer (NK) cells, which is actively involved in preventing metastasis and destroying small metastases."[37]

Many things can create the perfect storm of chronic stress, and it has a real effect on your brain, your nervous system, your organ function, your hormones and your ability to handle additional stressors, or to just enjoy life. It truly can lead to disease and even death! I'm not trying to be a drama queen, but learning what you need to navigate stress is one of the best things you can do for yourself. There is no life without stress, so we better learn how to manage it! This will look different for each and every one of us, but one thread that binds us is that we need genuine connection, to others and to ourselves! Exhale your worries away, if only for a moment, and let that oxytocin flow with your closest friends and family!

Mindfulness, a practice based in Buddhism that has woven its way into many forms of psychology and spirituality, is a proven avenue to treat stress. For thousands of years, humans have known that breath and being calm in the present moment can heal... especially if it is practiced enough to form a habit. In his book *Full Catastrophe Living*, Jon Kabat-Zin teaches readers how to embrace the inevitable chaos and intensity of life through simple, grounding techniques. There are many practitioners of mindfulness techniques out there, and one might be perfect for you! Books, videos, classes, in-person and on-line groups...you name it, people are getting their calm on!

So be free, dear humans, and help each other be free too! We certainly won't get to the end of our lives and regret being kind, to ourselves or others.

Remember my friends... we are AMAZING!

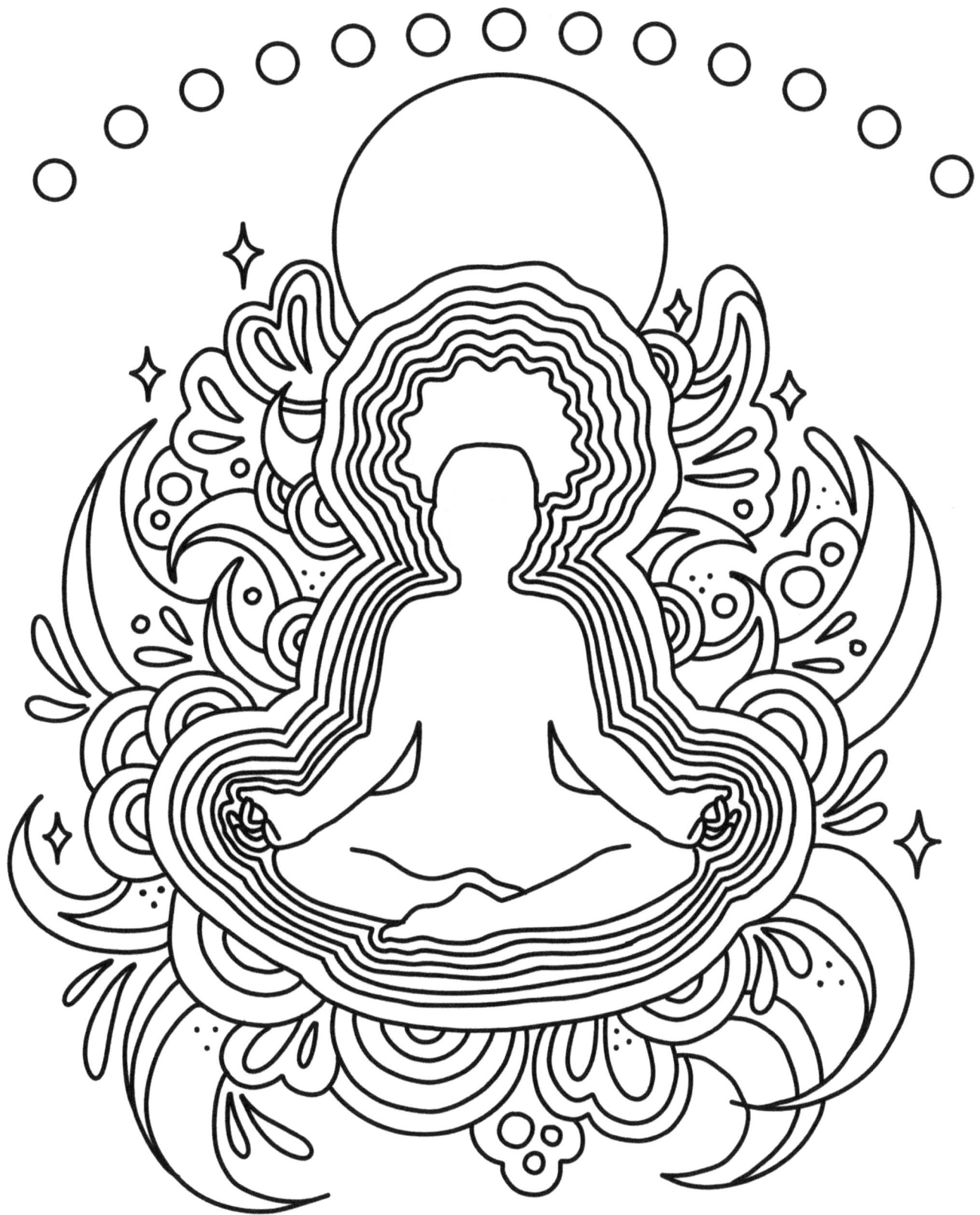

Glossary of Terms

Acid reflux: A condition where digestive juices go backwards up into the esophagus and irritate its lining. Also called 'heartburn'. Frequent episodes indicate GERD, or gastroesophageal reflux disease.

Adhesions: A situation in which the fascia in an area of the body sticks together, instead of sliding easily past each other. Similar to scar tissue, it restricts movement of structures that are supposed to move freely.

Adrenal fatigue: Not technically an accepted diagnosis by the allopathic medical community, the idea is that, after an extended period of stress where our adrenal glands are releasing cortisol and adrenaline, they start to get 'tired', which can result in general fatigue, difficulty sleeping or waking, and salt/sugar cravings. It is notable that fatigue is a symptom of many conditions, so make sure you are exploring all of the possibilities.

Allopathic: A term used to differentiate 'modern' medicine, whose remedies are commonly drugs and surgery, from other forms of medicine, such as acupuncture, herbalism, Ayurveda, and all realms of 'natural' medicine. In recent years, natural medicine is making its way into the allopathic world, creating a more holistic approach to health and healing.

Aorta: The aorta is an artery that carries blood away from the heart to all of the places it is needed in the body. The blood carried by the aorta is full of all of the components needed to nourish cells and their functions.

Arousal nonconcordance: The well-established phenomenon of a lack of overlap between how much blood is flowing to a person's genitals and how "turned on" they feel.

Asherman's syndrome: The formation of scar tissue inside the uterus, sometimes triggered by D&Cs, or abortions/terminations/evacuations. D&Cs may be performed to ensure all of the tissue is released following a miscarriage or childbirth, to remove polyps or other pathologies or to terminate an unwanted or unhealthy pregnancy (for an array of reasons).

Assigned female/male at birth (AFAB/AMAB): This is a way to acknowledge people who do not fit into the gender binary, and to make it clear that external genitalia fails to encompass the whole of us. Currently, we are assigned to one of three gender boxes at birth (female, male, intersex), but that label is problematic to many, and does not represent how we might later identify.

Blood cells: The main components of blood are plasma, red blood cells, white blood cells and platelets. Plasma is the liquid that blood cells float in. It is made up of water, antibodies, enzymes, salts and proteins. Red blood cells deliver oxygen to the whole body and collect carbon dioxide to be eliminated in the lungs. White blood cells are part of the body's immune system, as they help fight off pathogens. Platelets mainly exist to clot the blood, preventing you from losing too much blood and bleeding to death!

Body dysmorphia: The perception of oneself as physically flawed, to the point of real psychological distress. People with body dysmorphia are so hyper-focused on their perceived difference or flaw that it affects many aspects of life.

Cardiac output: The amount of blood the body pumps through its entire circulatory system in one minute. The average adult pumps 4.7 liters (5 quarts).

Cellular waste: The 'garbage' created by our cells as they perform their functions. Like all living things, our cells utilize the components they need, and discard the rest. Luckily, we have built-in systems to process and remove all of that rubbish!

Cervical fluid/mucus: A substance emitted from the cervix that changes in consistency during the course of a menstrual cycle. The thickness and viscosity varies from cottage-cheese-like to egg-white-like, depending on what the body is trying to achieve at the moment. Slippery, egg-white fluid is perfect to aid in sperm mobility, whereas thick fluid can inhibit it.

Cisgender: A person whose gender identity matches their sex assigned at birth.

Corpus luteum: This is the progesterone-emitting structure that was once the follicle or casing that contained the egg that ovulated in a given month. It will continue to release progesterone until menstruation, or in the event of a pregnancy, until the placenta takes over around 8-10 weeks after fertilization.

Digestive enzymes: Substances in the digestive tract that break down fats (lipase), carbohydrates (amylase) and proteins (proteases and peptidases).

Esophagus: Pathway from the throat to the stomach. A muscular tube.

Fascia: A thin and transparent but extremely strong connective tissue that covers each organ and muscle of the body and connects them in a web that allows individual movement but keeps the entire structure together. If you have ever prepared raw chicken, you have likely worked with it!

Gender dysphoria: The psychological distress one can experience at some point in their life if their gender identity does not match their sex assigned at birth.

GERD: Gastroesophageal reflux disease. A dysfunction of the sphincter between the esophagus and the stomach. Heartburn is a main symptom.

Gland: An organ in the body that secretes chemicals for use by many bodily functions.

Groups of muscles: While each muscle can perform a number of actions, muscle groups work together to enact more complex movements. Some common groupings are the rotator cuff (of the shoulder), the shoulder girdle and the pelvic girdle.

hCG (human chorionic gonadotropin): A hormone emitted by the first stage of a growing embryo and later by the placenta. It is what a pregnancy test detects. Some cancerous tumors also emit it, so it can indicate a growing tumor in the absence of a pregnancy.

Hiatal hernia: A hernia is when an organ or tissue protrudes through a muscle or fascia. It can happen over time or more quickly in the case of an injury. A hiatal hernia is when part of the stomach protrudes upwards through the diaphragm.

Holistic: A broad approach to health that incorporates multiple aspects of one's body, mind and spirit into the exploration of any health issues that arise. From looking at posture related to pain, to stress levels related to disease, it approaches the whole experience of a person instead of simply the area of pain or dysfunction.

Hormone: A substance released by body structures to stimulate specific cells to enact their roles in body function.

Hysterectomy: The removal of part or all of the womb. A total hysterectomy removes the uterus (including the cervix) and both ovaries and fallopian tubes. Sometimes, in partial hysterectomies, one or both ovaries and/or the cervix is left intact. If one or both ovaries remain, they will release the reproductive hormones that keep the body in balance for the remainder of the person's life. If they are removed, some sort of hormone replacement therapy is often utilized to reduce suffering and keep their hormones in balance. The cervix might be removed to prevent cervical cancer, but if it is not, it can prevent urinary issues from developing later.

Intersex: People born with chromosomal, genetic, hormonal and/or physical variations from the binary.

Ischial tuberosities: V-shaped bones at the bottom of the pelvis, aka the sitz/sit/sitting bones, as they are the bones you feel touching the surface sat upon. Many muscles attach to this area, both pelvic and leg muscles.

Lymphatic system: A network of fluid, vessels and nodes that function as a pathway for removing cellular waste and pathogens from the body. Working directly with the cardiovascular (blood) system, it draws fluid out of the blood in the magical space (aka capillary beds) between the arteries (blood moving away from your heart) and the veins (blood moving towards your heart) and cleans it. Any pathogens that can't be destroyed on the spot get taken to your lymph nodes to be destroyed. The cleaned-out fluid then goes back into the blood, maintaining just the right amount of pressure to keep all systems functioning optimally! Unlike the cardiovascular system which has a heart to pump the blood through the closed system, lymphatic fluid requires us to move to keep it going!

Marrow: The marrow is a gelatinous material in the center of our bones that contains our stem cells. Stem cells are immature cells and there are two types. One is red marrow (hematopoietic) and it forms our red and white blood cells. The other is yellow marrow (mesenchymal) and it forms our fat, cartilage and bone.

Mindfulness: The practice of bringing yourself into the present moment without judgement, or trying to change it.

Neurogastroenterology: The study of the nervous system of the gut. Includes the liver, pancreas and the gastrointestinal tract and encompasses control of digestion through the enteric nervous system (ENS), the central nervous system (CNS) and integrative centers in sympathetic ganglia. A relatively new area of study/specialty, scientists are exploring the many physical and psychological roles and effects of how well (or poorly) this system works.

Neuropeptide: Proteins produced by neurons that play a role in nerve conduction.

Nonbinary: More than two options. People who identify as nonbinary don't fit or support the limiting system that society has created by only presenting/accepting 'male' or 'female' as options of identity. This term has developed as a way to include more of the numerous ways people live and identify, and to recognize the expansive reality.

Pathogens/pathologies: Disease cells/diseases. A pathogen is a bacteria, virus or other microorganism that can cause a pathology, or disease.

Placenta: An organ that develops during pregnancy to support the life of a fetus. It attaches to the wall of the uterus and filters nutrients out of the blood, which it delivers through the umbilical cord to the fetus.

Precursors (hormone): A substance that is used to create a hormone.

Primal: Essential, basic. A primal need or fear is related to something we need to survive, or a threat to those needs.

Resorption: Reabsorption, specifically of cells or tissue into the circulatory system.

Scar tissue: The body's protective response to injury; cells and collagen that form over an injury. Because it needs to form quickly, it layers in irregular patterns, making the tissue strong and thicker than the surrounding tissue.

Sciatic nerve: A bundle of 5 nerve roots from the low back and sacrum, the sciatic nerve is the largest nerve in the body. Compression of this nerve can cause pain in the low back, SI joint, buttock, hip and down the leg.

Sex assigned at birth: Based on external genitalia. Does not always match the person's identity as they get older.

Sphincter: A ring of muscle at the opening (or closing) of a structure such as the anus, the urethra or the stomach. It contracts to close the opening and relaxes to open it.

Spinal compression: Due to injury or muscle tension, the vertebrae and discs compress, which can cause discomfort and pain. Chronic tension around the spine can make one more prone to bulging or herniated discs.

Spinal vertebrae: The bones of the spine, each designed to allow movement, cushioned by the intervertebral discs, and to protect the spinal cord, which connects the central nervous system to the peripheral nervous system.

Steroid hormones: Derived from cholesterol, this group of hormones (glucocorticoids, mineralocorticoids, androgens, estrogens and progestogens) are emitted from the adrenal cortex, the ovaries and testes, and the placenta.

Transgender: Someone whose gender identity does not match their sex assigned at birth.

Urogenital: Simply put, the urinary and genital systems! A specialty in allopathic medicine, as well as a closely related grouping of functions.

Vena cava (inferior and superior): The largest vein bringing deoxygenated blood from all of the other veins of the body to the lungs, where it can be reoxygenated and pumped back into the heart, before it goes for another round through the body!

Gratitude.

So much gratitude to my teachers and inspirators in all forms:

Rosita Arvigo, DN (and her beloved teachers Don Elijio Panti, Miss Hortence Robinson and Miss Juana, bush doctors and herbalist midwives of the Cayo District of Belize), Isa Herrera, PT, Tami Lynn Kent, PT, Lara Briden, ND, and all of my clients, wellness colleagues, helpers and friends.

A heartfelt thank you goes to the content competency advisors...you made this book better! Holly Grace Currie, Director of Youth & Prevention Services at: Haven Women's Center, Kelly Marshall, Educator at Transforming Wellness, Kristen Hayes, all-around badass, and Jean McCray for your encouragement and introducing me to the digital possibilities! And the copy-editing extraordinaires... Kris, Milly, Patricia and Celinda...thank goodness for you all!

A very special Hip-Hip-Hooray! goes to my dear friend and editor Abe Louise Young, whose personal and professional encouragement are just what I need, when I need it most! Thanks for the loving encouragement, and the detail-oriented experience, perspective and wisdom!

Lastly but profoundly, big love goes out to my mom, Celinda Ann Ranweiler Doyle, who taught me early the healing power of massage and the proper name for all of the body's parts! She is a nurse of nurses, and a mom of moms...and I am proud to know her!

Each one, teach one...as they say.

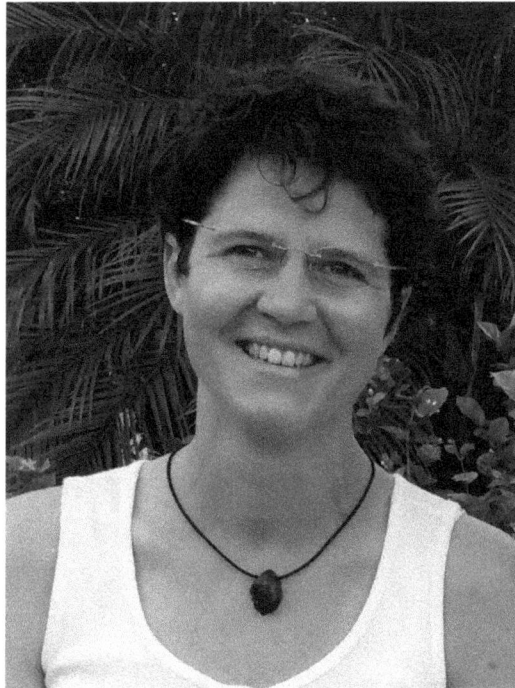

Rachael Wilder has been a massage therapist
in Austin TX since 2009, and has specialized
in abdominal and pelvic health since 2012.

Inspired by her clients' journeys with digestive and pelvic health,
including the emotional aspects of wellness, she created
The People's Pelvis to inspire others! While there is a lot to know
about pelvic health in all of our bodies, she wanted it to be fun,
inclusive and engaging. *The People's Pelvis* is all of that, and more!

Notes

*All note and reference links are published on the website,
www.peoplespelvis.com for easy clicking!

1. Lebrecht, James; Newnham, Nicole; Radcliff, David. Crip Camp. Film. Higher Ground Productions. 2020. *https://www.imdb.com/title/tt8923484/*

2. Aging Changes in the Bones-Muscles-Joints. Mount Sinai Health Library. Reviewed July, 2020. *https://www.mountsinai.org/health-library/special-topic/aging-changes-in-the-bones-muscles-joints*

3. Ojumah, Naomi; Loukas, Marios. The intriguing History of the Term Sacrum. Review. The Spine Scholar, vol 2 num 1, 2018. *https://static1.squarespace.com/static/554037b3e4b0da169013a32f/t/5c06f2141ae6cf9eac-24de4b/1543959060660/historyofsacrum_%281%29+%281%29.pdf*

4. Sattar MH, Guthrie ST. Anatomy, Back, Sacral Vertebrae. [Updated 2020 Jul 31]. In: StatPearls [Internet]. Treasure Island (FL): StatPearls Publishing; 2021 Jan-. Available from: *https://www.ncbi.nlm.nih.gov/books/NBK551653/*

5. Lichtenstein, Mia Beck et al. "Exercise addiction in adolescents and emerging adults - Validation of a youth version of the Exercise Addiction Inventory." Journal of behavioral addictions vol. 7,1 (2018): 117-125. doi:10.1556/2006.7.2018.01. *https://www.ncbi.nlm.nih.gov/pmc/articles/PMC6035018/*

6. Hererra, Isa. Female Pelvic Floor Training for Birth and Wellness Professionals. Pelvic Pain Relief. New York, NY 2017. *https://pelvicpainrelief.com/pelvicwellness/*

7. Nagoski, Emily. Come As You Are. Simon and Schuster, New York, 2015.

8. Bartosch, Jamie. Kegels: The 30-Second Exercise That Can Improve Incontinence and Sex. Interview. University of Chicago Medicine. October 2018. *https://www.uchicagomedicine.org/forefront/womens-health-articles/kegels-the-30-second-exercise-that-can-improve-incontinence-and-sex*

9. Koch, Liz. The Psoas Book. Guinea Pig Publications, Lawrence, KS, 1981. *https://coreawareness.com/product/the-psoas-book-new-30th-anniversary-revised-edition/*

10. Martínez-Hurtado I, Arguisuelas MD, Almela-Notari P, et al. Effects of diaphragmatic myofascial release on gastroesophageal reflux disease: a preliminary randomized controlled trial. Sci Rep. 2019;9(1):7273. Published 2019 May 13. doi:10.1038/s41598-019-43799-y. *https://www.nature.com/articles/s41598-019-43799-y*

11. Kinsinger, Sarah. How Breathing Exercises Relieve Stress and Improve Digestive Health. Loyola Medicine, December 15th, 2017. *https://loyolamedicine.org/blog/breathing-stress-improve-digestive*

12. Pinched (compressed) Nerve. WebMD. Reviewed by Ambardakar, Nayana, MD. September 1st, 2020. *https://www.webmd.com/pain-management/guide/compressed-nerves*

13. Kiff, E.S., Barnes, P.R.H., Swash, M. Evidence of Pudendal Neuropathy in Patients with Perineal Descent and Chronic Straining at Stool. Gut, 25, 1279-1282. Saint Mark's Hospital, London, 1984. *https://www.ncbi.nlm.nih.gov/pmc/articles/PMC1432308/*

14. Bonaz B, Sinniger V, Pellissier S. The Vagus Nerve in the Neuro-Immune Axis: Implications in the Pathology of the Gastrointestinal Tract. Front Immunol. 2017 Nov 2;8:1452. doi: 10.3389/fimmu.2017.01452. PMID: 29163522; PMCID: PMC5673632. *https://pubmed.ncbi.nlm.nih.gov/29163522/*

15. Zimmerman, Edith. "I now suspect the Vagus Nerve as the Key to Wellbeing". Science of Us. The Cut, May 2019. *https://www.thecut.com/2019/05/i-now-suspect-the-vagus-nerve-is-the-key-to-well-being.html*

16. Bergland, Christopher. Longer Exhalations Are an Easy Way to Hack Your Vagus Nerve. Stress. Psychology Today, May 19th, 2019. *https://www.psychologytoday.com/us/blog/the-athletes-way/201905/longer-exhalations-are-easy-way-hack-your-vagus-nerve*

17. Ford, Heather Flint, OD. Seeing Blue: The Impact of Excessive Blue Light Exposure. Review of Optometry, April 15th, 2016. *https://www.reviewofoptometry.com/article/seeing-blue-the-impact-of-excessive-blue-light-exposure*

18. Choudhuri, Alpana and Murari. Hormones and Neurotransmitters: The Differences and Curious Similarities. The Biochemists, June 26th, 2018. *https://medium.com/the-biochemists/hormones-and-neurotransmitters-the-differences-and-curious-similarities-46c6095b825*

19. Gaskin, Ina May. Ina May's Guide to Childbirth. Bantam Books, May 4th, 2003.

20. Whitehead, Christina. Ligaments of the Female Reproductive Tract. Teach Me Anatomy, January 2th, 2020. *https://teachmeanatomy.info/pelvis/female-reproductive-tract/ligaments/*

21. Taylor, Sonya Renee. The Body is Not An Apology. Berrett-Koehler Publishers; 1st edition February 13, 2018.

22. Yaribeygi, Habib et al. "The impact of stress on body function: A review." EXCLI journal vol. 16 1057-1072. 21 Jul. 2017, doi:10.17179/excli2017-480. *https://www.ncbi.nlm.nih.gov/pmc/articles/PMC5579396/*

23. Remoundou K, Koundouri P. Environmental effects on public health: an economic perspective. Int J Environ Res Public Health. 2009;6(8):2160-2178. doi:10.3390/ijerph6082160. *https://www.ncbi.nlm.nih.gov/pmc/articles/PMC2738880/*

24. Olsen, Natalie R.D., L.D., ACSM EP-C. What to Eat and What to Avoid If You Have Endometriosis. Healthline, April 17th, 2020. *https://www.healthline.com/health/endometriosis/endometriosis-diet*

25. Jahanfar, Shayesteh. "Genetic and environmental determinants of menstrual characteristics." Indian journal of human genetics vol. 18,2 (2012): 187-92. doi:10.4103/0971-6866.100759. *https://www.ncbi.nlm.nih.gov/pmc/articles/PMC3491292/*

26. Felson, Sabrina MD (Reviewed by). Adhesions, General and After Surgery. WebMD, June 2nd, 2020. *https://www.webmd.com/a-to-z-guides/adhesion-general-post-surgery*

27. Pastore, Elizabeth A, and Wendy B Katzman. "Recognizing myofascial pelvic pain in the female patient with chronic pelvic pain." Journal of obstetric, gynecologic, and neonatal nursing : JOGNN vol. 41,5 (2012): 680-91. doi:10.1111/j.1552-6909.2012.01404.x. *https://www.ncbi.nlm.nih.gov/pmc/articles/PMC3492521/*

28. Mays, Vickie M et al. "Race, race-based discrimination, and health outcomes among African Americans." Annual review of psychology vol. 58 (2007): 201-25. doi:10.1146/annurev.psych.57.102904.190212. *https://www.ncbi.nlm.nih.gov/pmc/articles/PMC4181672/*

29. Martin, Robert D. "The Macho Sperm Myth". Aeon, August 23rd, 2018. *https://aeon.co/essays/the-idea-that-sperm-race-to-the-egg-is-just-another-macho-myth*

30. Telfer, Nicole. "What's 'Normal'?: Menstrual Cycle Length and Variation." Clue, February 1st, 2021. *https://helloclue.com/articles/cycle-a-z/what's-normal-menstrual-cycle-length-and-variation*

31. Netter, Frank H. Atlas of Human Anatomy. Philadelphia, PA : Saunders/Elsevier, 2011. Plate 366.

32. Rey R, Josso N, Racine C. Sexual Differentiation. [Updated 2020 May 27]. In: Feingold KR, Anawalt B, Boyce A, et al., editors. Endotext [Internet]. South Dartmouth (MA): MDText.com, Inc.; 2000-. Available from: *https://www.ncbi.nlm.nih.gov/books/NBK279001/*

33. Harden, K Paige, and Kelly L Klump. "Introduction to the special issue on gene-hormone interplay." Behavior genetics vol. 45,3 (2015): 263-7. doi:10.1007/s10519-015-9717-7. *https://www.ncbi.nlm.nih.gov/pmc/articles/PMC4445642/*

34. Dotto, Gian-Paolo. "Gender and sex-time to bridge the gap." EMBO molecular medicine vol. 11,5 (2019): e10668. doi:10.15252/emmm.201910668. *https://www.ncbi.nlm.nih.gov/pmc/articles/PMC6505576/*

35. InterACT: Advocates for Intersex Youth. FAQ: What is Intersex? InterAct: Advocates for Intersex Youth, Sudbury, MA. Updated May 18th, 2020. *https://interactadvocates.org/faq/*

36. What Are STD's? STD's. Planned Parenthood. 2020. *https://www.plannedparenthood.org/learn/stds-hiv-safer-sex*

37. Salleh, Mohd Razali. "Life event, stress and illness." The Malaysian journal of medical sciences : MJMS vol. 15,4 (2008): 9-18. *https://www.ncbi.nlm.nih.gov/pmc/articles/PMC3341916/*

References

Aging Changes in the Bones-Muscles-Joints. Mount Sinai Health Library. Reviewed July, 2020. *https://www.mountsinai.org/health-library/special-topic/aging-changes-in-the-bones-muscles-joints*

Antoniou-Tsigkos A, **Zapanti E**, Ghizzoni L, et al. **Adrenal Androgens.** [Updated 2019 Jan 5]. In: Feingold KR, Anawalt B, Boyce A, et al., editors. Endotext [Internet]. South Dartmouth (MA): MDText.com, Inc.; 2000-. Available from: *www.ncbi.nlm.nih.gov/books/NBK278929/*

Bartosch, Jamie. **Kegels: The 30-Second Exercise That Can Improve Incontinence and Sex.** Interview. University of Chicago Medicine. October 2018. *https://www.uchicagomedicine.org/forefront/womens-health-articles/kegels-the-30-second-exercise-that-can-improve-incontinence-and-sex*

Bergland, Christopher. **Longer Exhalations Are an Easy Way to Hack Your Vagus Nerve.** Stress. Psychology Today, May 19th, 2019. *https://www.psychologytoday.com/us/blog/the-athletes-way/201905/longer-exhalations-are-easy-way-hack-your-vagus-nerve*

Bonaz B, **Sinniger** V, **Pellissier** S. **The Vagus Nerve in the Neuro-Immune Axis: Implications in the Pathology of the Gastrointestinal Tract.** Front Immunol. 2017 Nov 2;8:1452. doi: 10.3389/fimmu.2017.01452. PMID: 29163522; PMCID: PMC5673632. *https://pubmed.ncbi.nlm.nih.gov/29163522/*

Briden, Lara. **The Period Repair Manual.** Australia: Macmillan, 2018.

Choudhuri, Alpana and Murari. **Hormones and Neurotransmitters: The Differences and Curious Similarities**. The Biochemists, June 26, 2018. *https://medium.com/the-biochemists/hormones-and-neurotransmitters-the-differences-and-curious-similarities-46c6095b825*

Cuncic, Arlin. **How Hormones Play a Role in Social Anxiety.** Mental Health A-Z. Very Well Mind. 2020. *https://www.verywellmind.com/effect-of-hormones-on-social-anxiety-4129255.*

Dotto, Gian-Paolo. **"Gender and sex-time to bridge the gap."** EMBO molecular medicine vol. 11,5 (2019): e10668. doi:10.15252/emmm.201910668. *https://www.ncbi.nlm.nih.gov/pmc/articles/PMC6505576/*

Felson, Sabrina MD (Reviewed by). **Adhesions, General and After Surgery.** WebMD, June 2nd, 2020. *https://www.webmd.com/a-to-z-guides/adhesion-general-post-surgery*

Ford, Heather Flint, OD. **Seeing Blue: The Impact of Excessive Blue Light Exposure**. Review of Optometry, April 15, 2016. *https://www.reviewofoptometry.com/article/seeing-blue-the-impact-of-excessive-blue-light-exposure*

Hererra, Isa. **Female Pelvic Floor Training for Birth and Wellness Professionals.** Pelvic Pain Relief. New York, NY 2017. *https://pelvicpainrelief.com/pelvicwellness/*

INPHA Nutraceuticals: Male Urogenital System Disorders. Pathologies. 2015-2020. *https://www.inpha.it/en-us/Pathologies/Detail/ArticleID/27/Male-urogenital-system-diseases*

InterACT: Advocates for Intersex Youth. FAQ: What is Intersex? Updated May 18th, 2020. *https://interactadvocates.org/faq/*

Harden, K Paige, and Kelly L **Klump**. **"Introduction to the special issue on gene-hormone interplay."** *Behavior genetics* vol. 45,3 (2015): 263-7. doi:10.1007/s10519-015-9717-7. *https://www.ncbi.nlm.nih.gov/pmc/articles/PMC4445642/*

Jahanfar, Shayesteh. **"Genetic and environmental determinants of menstrual characteristics."** *Indian journal of human genetics* vol. 18,2 (2012): 187-92. doi:10.4103/0971-6866.100759. *https://www.ncbi.nlm.nih.gov/pmc/articles/PMC3491292/*

Kent, Tami. **Wild Feminine.** Atria Books/Beyond Words, 2011.

Kiff, E.S., **Barnes**, P.R.H., **Swash**, M. **Evidence of Pudendal Neuropathy in Patients with Perineal Descent and Chronic Straining at Stool.** Gut, **25**, 1279-1282. Saint Mark's Hospital, London, 1984. *https://www.ncbi.nlm.nih.gov/pmc/articles/PMC1432308/*

Kinsinger, Sarah. **How Breathing exercises Relieve Stress and Improve Digestive Health.** Loyola Medicine, December 15th, 2017. *https://loyolamedicine.org/blog/breathing-stress-improve-digestive*

Koch, Liz. **The Psoas Book.** Guinea Pig Publications, Lawrence, KS, 1981. *https://coreawareness.com/product/the-psoas-book-new-30th-anniversary-revised-edition/*

Lebrecht, James; **Newnham**, Nicole; **Radcliff**, David. **Crip Camp.** Film. Higher Ground Productions. 2020. *https://www.imdb.com/title/tt8923484/*

Lichtenstein, Mia Beck et al. "**Exercise addiction in adolescents and emerging adults - Validation of a youth version of the Exercise Addiction Inventory.**" *Journal of behavioral addictions* vol. 7,1 (2018): 117-125. doi:10.1556/2006.7.2018.01. *https://www.ncbi.nlm.nih.gov/pmc/articles/PMC6035018/*

Martin, Robert D. "**The Macho Sperm Myth**". Aeon, August 23rd, 2018. *https://aeon.co/essays/the-idea-that-sperm-race-to-the-egg-is-just-another-macho-myth*

Martínez-Hurtado I, Arguisuelas MD, **Almela-Notari** P, et al. **Effects of diaphragmatic myofascial release on gastroesophageal reflux disease:** a preliminary randomized controlled trial. Sci Rep. 2019;9(1):7273. Published 2019 May 13. doi:10.1038/s41598-019-43799-y. *https://www.nature.com/articles/s41598-019-43799-y*

Mays, Vickie M et al. "**Race, race-based discrimination, and health outcomes among African Americans.**" Annual review of psychology vol. 58 (2007): 201-25. doi:10.1146/annurev.psych.57.102904.190212. *https://www.ncbi.nlm.nih.gov/pmc/articles/PMC4181672/*

McLeod, Saul. **What Is the Stress Response?** Biological Psychology. Simple Psychology, 2010. *https://www.simplypsychology.org/stress-biology.html*

Nagoski, Emily. **Come As You Are.** Simon and Schuster, 2015.

Netter, Frank H. **Atlas of Human Anatomy.** Philadelphia, PA : Saunders/Elsevier, 2011.

Ojumah, Naomi; **Loukas**, Marios. **The intriguing History of the Term Sacrum.** Review. The Spine Scholar, vol 2 num 1, 2018. *https://static1.squarespace.com/static/554037b3e4b0da169013a32f/t/5c06f2141ae6cf9eac-24de4b/1543959060660/historyofsacrum_%281%29+%281%29.pdf*

Olsen, Natalie R.D., L.D., ACSM EP-C. **What to Eat and What to Avoid If You Have Endometriosis.** Healthline, April 17th, 2020. *https://www.healthline.com/health/endometriosis/endometriosis-diet*

Pastore, Elizabeth A, and Wendy B **Katzman.** "**Recognizing myofascial pelvic pain in the female patient with chronic pelvic pain.**" *Journal of obstetric, gynecologic, and neonatal nursing : JOGNN* vol. 41,5 (2012): 680-91. doi:10.1111/j.1552-6909.2012.01404.x. *https://www.ncbi.nlm.nih.gov/pmc/articles/PMC3492521/*

Pinched (compressed) Nerve. WebMD. Reviewed by **Ambardakar**, Nayana, MD. September 1st, 2020. *https://www.webmd.com/pain-management/guide/compressed-nerves*

Ponny Fights For Honest Sex Education. Advocates for Youth: Young, Powerful, Taking Over. 2020. *https://advocatesforyouth.org/issue/honest-sex-education/*

Ramanathan, Mangalam. **Hormones and chemicals Linked with Our Emotions.** Amrita Vishwa Vidyapeetham. 2018. *https://www.amrita.edu/news/hormones-and-chemicals-linked-our-emotion*

Remoundou K, **Koundouri** P. **Environmental effects on public health: an economic perspective.** Int J Environ Res Public Health. 2009;6(8):2160-2178. doi:10.3390/ijerph6082160. *https://www.ncbi.nlm.nih.gov/pmc/articles/PMC2738880/*

Rey R, Josso N, **Racine** C. **Sexual Differentiation.** [Updated 2020 May 27]. In: Feingold KR, Anawalt B, Boyce A, et al., editors. Endotext [Internet]. South Dartmouth (MA): MDText.com, Inc.; 2000-. Available from: *https://www.ncbi.nlm.nih.gov/books/NBK279001/*

Rifkin, Rachael; **How Shallow Breathing Affects Your Whole Body.** Health. Headspace, 2017. *https://www.headspace.com/blog/2017/08/15/shallow-breathing-whole-body/*

Salleh, Mohd Razali. **"Life Event, Stress and Illness."** The Malaysian journal of medical sciences : MJMS vol. 15,4 (2008): 9-18. https://www.ncbi.nlm.nih.gov/pmc/articles/PMC3341916/

Sattar MH, **Guthrie** ST. **Anatomy, Back, Sacral Vertebrae.** [Updated 2020 Jul 31]. In: StatPearls [Internet]. Treasure Island (FL): StatPearls Publishing; 2021 Jan-. Available from: *https://www.ncbi.nlm.nih.gov/books/NBK551653/*

Singer, Katie. **Garden of Fertility.** Avery, 2004.

Soran H, Wu FC. **Endocrine causes of erectile dysfunction.** Int J Androl. 2005 Dec;28 Suppl 2:28-34. doi: 10.1111/j.1365-2605.2005.00596.x. PMID: 16236061. *https://pubmed.ncbi.nlm.nih.gov/16236061/*

Taylor, Sonya Renee. **The Body is Not An Apology.** Berrett-Koehler Publishers; 1st edition February 13, 2018.

Teach Consent. Ask, Listen. Respect. Virginia Sexual & Domestic Violence Action Alliance. *http://storage.cloversites.com/virginiasexualdomesticviolenceactionallianc/documents/Facilitator%20discussion%20guide%202018-FINAL.pdf*

Telfer, Nicole. **"What's 'Normal'?: Menstrual Cycle Length and Variation."** Clue, February 1st, 2021. *https://helloclue.com/articles/cycle-a-z/what's-normal-menstrual-cycle-length-and-variation*

Turley, Raymond Kent; **Spinal Cord Compression.** Health Encyclopedia. University of Rochester Medical Center, 2002. *https://www.urmc.rochester.edu/encyclopedia/content.aspx?ContentTypeID=134&ContentID=13*

Weschler, Toni. **Taking Charge of Your Fertility.** William Morrow Paperbacks, July, 2015.

What Are STD's? STD's. Planned Parenthood. 2020. *https://www.plannedparenthood.org/learn/stds-hiv-safer-sex*

Whitehead, Christina. **Ligaments of the Female Reproductive Tract.** Teach Me Anatomy, January 2th, 2020. *https://teachmeanatomy.info/pelvis/female-reproductive-tract/ligaments/*

Wu, Katherine. **"Love Actually: The Science Behind Lust, Attraction and Companionship."** Blog. Harvard University, 2017. *http://sitn.hms.harvard.edu/flash/2017/love-actually-science-behind-lust-attraction-companionship/*

Yaribeygi, Habib et al. **"The Impact of Stress on Body Function: A Review."** EXCLI journal vol. 16 1057-1072. 21 Jul. 2017, doi:10.17179/excli2017-480. *https://www.ncbi.nlm.nih.gov/pmc/articles/PMC5579396/*

Zimmerman, Edith. **"I now suspect the Vagus Nerve as the Key to Wellbeing."** Science of Us. The Cut, May 2019. *https://www.thecut.com/2019/05/i-now-suspect-the-vagus-nerve-is-the-key-to-well-being.html*

www.ingramcontent.com/pod-product-compliance
Lightning Source LLC
Chambersburg PA
CBHW042353030426
42336CB00029B/3470